The Mariachis Are Gone

The Mariachis Are Gone

The true story of how Alzheimer's disease tests a love. Told with pathos and black humor.

By Lois Cowan Rische

Cover design by F. Cowan
Editor, F. Cowan

International Standard Book Number: 0-9663971-0-X

Library of Congress Catalog Card Number: 98-91330

Manufactured in the United States of America
By
D. Armstrong Book Printing Company, Inc.

A portion of the profits from this book
will be donated to The Alzheimer's Association

Dedication
To

My daughters, Fontaine and Susan, who listened every day, as these writings progressed.

And to my son, Michael, who introduced me to the computer and made my life easier.

And to my friends, Dot Dimiero and Dana Aichler. They inspired and urged me to write this book.

This is a true story, where the names have been changed to protect the innocent. For the sake of the story, it has been only very slightly fictionalized.

THE MARIACHIS ARE GONE
A Story of Commitment

"I have you fast in my fortress.
And will not let you depart.
But put you down into the dungeon
In the round-tower of my heart.

And there will I keep you forever.
Yes, forever and a day.
Till the wall shall crumble to ruin.
And molder in dust away."

From "The Children's Hour" by Henry Wadsworth Longfellow.

Table of Contents

Acknowledgements

My special thanks to Claudia Kolker, staff reporter for the Houston Chronicle. Ms. Kolker, while a reporter for the Houston Press, launched this book when she did an in depth story of "The Mariachis Are Gone." (*Houston Press* cover story August 3, 1995).

THE COLONEL

I had been told that Colonel Becker had been cooling his heels for more than an hour in the waiting room. This was The University of Texas, Department of Ophthalmology's Clinic in Galveston, Texas. The colonel was to see me for an eye exam. There had been a scheduling error at the front appointment desk, so things were out of kilter.

With a small amount of trepidation, I approached the waiting room. It was easy to pick out my patient. Colonel Becker sat very erect. He was a striking-looking man. Even in his Sears Roebuck-style clothes, with the too-short pants, he stood out. However, his cowboy boots were not Sears' best. They looked expensive, hand-made, and had a high spit shine. He looked very Aryan, with pinkish skin and steel gray eyes. His jaw was set like that of an executioner. His whole demeanor screamed "Texas." Surely, his horse was tied up out front.

Later I learned that he had driven from Houston, a distance of about fifty miles, and had been on the island since very early for a fasting blood sugar test. I apologized for the wait. He hadn't eaten since dinner time yesterday. It was now past noon.

I took a brief history. His answers were short and terse. If ever I saw a man on the verge of a growl, he was it. He had to be mean. I asked him to sit in the examining chair. He did so, without a wasted motion. With a little bit of disgust about the cowboy's attitude, and in order to move my examining stool, I kicked it gently. It rolled to rest just where I wanted it, right in front of the colonel. As a matter of fact it rolled right up next to, and touching, his precious cowboy boots. "Whoa . . . there, lady, aren't you getting just a little bit obstreperous?" And he smiled an infectious half-smile.

I presented him with the first test. He put on the red-and-green glasses. I held a flashlight containing four lighted red-and-green dots. I asked him, "What do you see?"

"Hamburgers," he replied. We laughed. Then, slowly, and with the utmost sincerity, and in an authentic Texas drawl, he said, "You're beautiful." His eyes sparkled and his face was like a whole new world. Moments seemed to pass as I accepted his compliment in silence.

He said he would find it very difficult to continue with the examination without lunch. Suddenly, he was offering to take me to lunch, anywhere on the island. Don't ask me why, but for some reason I went with him.

There was no horse tied up outside, only a dusty old, non-descript brown Toyota with a Texas A & M decal that was upside down and backwards on the rear window. The car looked and smelled like a working ranch car. And how odd, I mused, why on earth would he have a telephone in a car like this? Oh well . . . the telephone was also brown.

Since arriving in Texas, almost two decades ago, I had never come to know an Aggie really well. Aggies were enigmas. In Texas, they are the butt of an enormous repertoire of stupid jokes. Certainly, he was a member of the world's largest non-paying fraternity. Founded in 1876, the school quickly rose to academic prominence. Once an Aggie, always an Aggie. Their loyalties are fierce. And now, I was about to make my acquaintance with an Aggie, up close and personal.

I suggested Gaido's for lunch, the nicest seafood restaurant in Galveston. It was just a few minutes away, down on the seawall. We had a lovely, fun, two-hour lunch. We barely scratched our past lives, and covered only the essential biographic information: I was a widow with three children. He was a widower. (Later, he confessed that he was really a divorcee, and his ex-wife was deceased). Also, he had seven children.

I learned that he had lived with his family in the Washington, D.C. area at the same time that I had been living just a stone's throw away in Maryland. At the time, I had been eleven years old and in the sixth grade. He had been thirtyish, with one child and twins on the way, and was working in military intelligence at the Pentagon.

Now, I refer to his style of eating as, "in military fashion." Sitting erect and very tall, he rearranged almost everything on the table. When the food arrived, he straightened it on the plate and shoveled it into neat little mounds. Then, silently and carefully, he ate one thing at a time until it was gone. This was interrupted only with a little procedure that he did for me, and was a preview of things to come. He insisted on buttering my bread, which he did with the same exactness, with the same focus. I felt a tinge of, "I'm perfectly capable of buttering my own bread." Nevertheless, I felt an indescribable feeling of being with a man who knew just how to take care of a woman, and what's more, he loved doing it. That was not all bad.

A wave of feeling passed over me, a feeling that I could not identify, and in the months to come it would become recurrent in me. Silently, we lingered over our coffee, longer than we should have. We watched the festive surreys, with red-and-white canopies, and the laughing occupants pedaling by.

We watched, and felt the rhythm of the waves, as we gazed out onto the Gulf of Mexico . . . and our souls sang silent songs.

We returned to my clinic. Two brochures on my desk got his attention. I was on the verge of building a harpsichord (from a kit) and was trying to make the final selection. This launched a fifteen minute discussion on high-fidelity music components and our mutual interest in music and electronics.

"I've never met a woman who built a Heathkit," he said as he looked at me in amazement.

I said, "Crazy, isn't it? Now you have. Now let's get to work."

During the exam my mind drifted back to lunch and the bread-buttering ritual. I was taken with the man's incredible hands. They were large and muscular, and hairy, and rough with brown spots. The knuckles were knobby and the veins prominent. They looked as if he had spent much of his life working in the fields. They were fine.

I took a deep breath. Throughout the coming years my fascination with his hands remained with me. Later I would do a photographic study of them.

The exam was complete. Very matter-of-factly, Colonel Becker said he would like to see me again. He said he was very busy with his paging business, and would have to be in Washington, meeting with the F.C.C. attorneys in the coming weeks. Curiously, he gave me three of his business cards and said, "If you don't hear from me in one month, I hope you will call me because I really do want to see you again. I mean that." He departed, slowly turning, with a twinkle in his eye, and a slow winding smile.

That night I had dinner at home in Houston with an old friend, Dorothy Coates. I told her, "I had a very interesting patient today, a retired army colonel who also has his own paging business in Houston. He was a bit of a cowboy, but at the same time, a gentleman, a real old-fashioned gentleman. His manners were impeccable. He's really much too old for me, though. He's sixty-four, and will be on Medicare next year. Oh well, it really doesn't matter, because I doubt that I'll ever see him again."

Recently, I had been dating a cardiovascular surgeon who was here from Cairo, working with Dr. Denton Cooley. He was a colonel in the reserve Egyptian army. Over the course of our six-month relationship, it became evident that we were not made for each other. In fact, under close scrutiny, I discovered that he was downright uncivilized. Most especially, his table manners were remarkable. They were gross. There was that last, unforgettable spaghetti dinner, which made the Egyptian history. That was one week previous to meeting the current colonel. Funny, isn't it, how timing can make the difference?

More than a month had passed since the colonel and I had lunched in Galveston. It was a Saturday morning when a friend called to offer me a couple of tickets to an Irish play at the Alley Theater. Having no men in my life, I called several girlfriends. It was rather late to be asking, and they all had previous plans. Suddenly I remembered Colonel Becker's cards and rustled in my purse and came up with one of them.. After I located the card, it took about fifteen minutes before I could muster the courage to dial his number. In my generation, it was still socially unacceptable to ring a man up on the telephone. Could I really do it?

The telephone rang and rang . . . and when I was on the verge of hanging up, a breathless Colonel Becker answered. He had been mowing the grass. I extended the theater invitation. He said he'd love to, but would have to call me back in a couple of hours to give me an answer because he was having an irregular heartbeat.

"For the love of God, Montessor," I thought, "What in hell are you doing out mowing the grass? Are you crazy? Don't you have any common sense at all? MEN!" I was appalled by his nonchalant attitude.

But I only said, "Don't you think it might be a good thing for you to save the grass for another day, and go inside and rest awhile with a cool drink ?"

The conversation really rattled me, disconcerting, to say the least. In exactly two hours he called back to say that his heartbeat had been restored to normal, he felt fine, and would be delighted to accept the theater invitation. He asked if I would be his guest for dinner at the Houston Club, before the theater. Of course I would.

He called for me at the appointed time, six, straight up. As we stepped out onto the front courtyard, in true military fashion, he offered me his arm on the way to the car.

It brought to mind the carefree days of the late forties, when I used to "drag" at The United States Naval Academy in Annapolis, Maryland. I used to walk the streets of that town, with my arm very proudly entwined with the arm of some good-looking midshipman.

They were all great-looking, perfectly wonderful, in their summer whites, or their winter blues. Either way, they were impressive.

That same feeling returned, the feeling I had gotten on the arms of the midshipmen, or more recently, the feeling that had come over me in the restaurant when I looked on as he buttered my bread. It was still not identifiable.

The Houston Club was the oldest gentlemen's club in Houston and was founded in 1894. It was the same as always, very nice, quiet and with the best of food, served unobtrusively. All of the employees greeted him enthusiastically. The club was within walking distance of his old office at The Federal Building and he had lunched there often, for many years. Earl, the tall Afro-American headwaiter, whose income tax Fritz used to do as a favor, was especially pleased to see him. They had known each other for about twenty-five years.

I wasn't accustomed to drinking a great deal, but since he ordered a Manhattan on-the-rocks, I thought a martini on-the-rocks might be appropriate. After two or three of those killer drinks, dinner was served. We had some great sirloin strips. Earl took a trip to the wine cellar and presented us with a bottle of Dom Perignon.

Their gingerbread is famous, and they keep the recipe secret. Fritz, very carefully, buttered a piece and handed it across the table to me. Midway through dinner Fritz suggested that he telephone the theater and try to exchange the tickets for the following night. That accomplished, we dined on for several more hours, finished the bottle of wine, and danced to some wonderful nineteen-forties and fifties piano music. The pianist had the longest fingers I'd ever seen. His name was Gibbons, father of Billy Gibbons, of "ZZ Top." Fritz finished with a Remy Martin.

After dinner, Fritz sat with his hands clasped, elbows resting on the table. From his expression I gleaned that he was evaluating me. He was. "Sweetheart, you're just beautiful . . . and I'm a lucky son-of-a-gun to have stumbled upon you. Most especially, I like that devilish air about you . . . and you're an independent woman. I don't believe I've ever known an independent woman, and to tell you the truth, it scares the hell out of me." We laughed and laughed.

When I arose from the table, I discovered that I definitely needed a strong military arm to hang onto. I hadn't felt this way since after football games, at the fraternity parties at the University of Maryland and the University of Virginia. "Oh God, be with me and with my spirit . . . I shall make it . . . Deo gratis."

On the way home he asked if I would like to go to his place for a demonstration of his Klipschorn speakers. That seemed agreeable. It was a clear, bright and balmy April night, and I thought . . . “a night with a thousand eyes.” It seemed a perfect evening, even in the dusty brown Toyota. I laid my head back. I began to feel not so good . . . like sick, sick, sick. I rolled down the window, and was just about blown away. Great Caesar’s Ghost! As I glanced across at the instrument panel, I saw we were edging past eighty-five miles per hour.

We arrived. Oh yes, unmistakably, we were in suburbia. I didn’t see many trees, just one-story houses that looked very much alike. It seemed there was a pickup truck or camper in every driveway. Somehow, this man seemed incongruous with this scene. Oh, well.

We were greeted by three yapping dogs. There were two miniature Chihuahuas and a West Highland terrier. I never could stand noisy pip-squeak dogs. The main room was small and dark. (He called it a den. Don’t you just hate it?) I have a visual knack of taking everything in, in a glance. There was split-pea-colored, sculpted wall-to-wall carpeting.

The furniture was difficult to classify. I later learned that most of it came from federal government auctions. There was a large, heavily-carved camphor oriental chest that was beautiful. Also, there was a collection of Indonesian wood carvings that was very nice.

Sitting alongside the carvings were a dozen or so bowling trophies. And, sure enough . . . there were the Klipschorns . . . in all their glory.

He put on a record by Ella Fitzgerald and we listened to all those wonderful songs, “Mr. Paganini,” “When I Take My Sugar To Tea,” “A Tisket A Tasket,” “Bess, You Is My Woman,” and many more.

I became sicker and sicker, and clammy and faint, and wished I wasn’t there. Suddenly, I vomited all over the green-sculpted carpeting.

As he assisted me to the bedroom, I reminded myself that this was our first date. He pulled back the covers on the king-sized bed, and laid me carefully down. I was silenced by my sickness, and mortified to think that I was even there at all, but feeling too bad to consciously care.

He took charge of the situation in a directive-type way. "You're too sick to drive home," he said. I voted by silent assent. With that, he cleaned up all the mess that stretched from here to kingdom come, put me into a pair of his pajamas, and brought me a pan.

For several hours he tended me with cold packs to my head. Then he brought out a precious little Martin ukulele which he played and sang the sweetest songs to me in an endearing tenor voice.

As I was serenaded by this most unusual man, I remember thinking that I was in a strange place with a strange man...and in spite of this, I felt very comfortable and very safe. As I dozed off, the soothing strains of several wonderful little tunes came to me, "Imagination, that's funny," and "Jada, Jada, Jada Jada Jing, Jing, Jing." And I remembered my father singing those same songs . . . while he strummed his banjo.

"TIJUANA BRASS"

I awakened at seven o'clock, and didn't feel so hot. My God, I was in men's pajamas on a large unfamiliar bed. And most disturbing was the condition of the other side of the bed. It was rumpled, and definitely had been slept in. I was horrified. I smelled bacon and eggs. There was some peppy music coming from the front of the house. "Tijuana Brass,". . . oh Jesus, that was it! Given the condition of my head, it was *not* a soothing sound. I wondered if he had any Chopin. Later, I figured out that this was his way of extricating me from the bed.

God, I must be in enemy territory. There were guns everywhere, propped against the wall. Well, a dozen or so at least. Was he a soldier of fortune? I wasn't at all acquainted with firearms, so I can't tell you what kinds of guns they were. Oh God, how am I going to get out of this one?

It was a small dark room with a dresser, a chest, a desk and a bedside table. There were tall piles of "Playboy" magazine, "National Geographic" and "Soviet Life." There were bookcases over the desk, with an assortment of books on the military, on weapons and brainwashing. I noticed such titles as "The Office of Strategic Services," "Photography," "World War II," "Asia," "Voodoo," "Head Hunters," and a myriad of books on intelligence, and Russia. There was, "The Devils of Loudun," by Aldous Huxley, "Witchcraft in France and Switzerland," "The Passive Aggressive Personality," "The

Criminal Mind," "The Craft of Intelligence," by Allen Dulles, "The World Bank," "Walden," by Thoreau, "Common Sense," by Thomas Paine, A Merriam Webster Dictionary, a Malay dictionary, one of Carl Sagan's books, "The Ascent of Man" and a "Roget's Thesaurus." There were only a few pieces of fiction; "The Robe," "Gone With The Wind," and two novels by John Fowles, "The Magus," and "The French Lieutenant's Woman." I made the assumption that the man was literate. I felt in a private surreptitious space. A wave of discordance welled up in my soul, but it was accompanied by an equally strong wave of curiosity, for which I felt an urgent need to satisfy.

There were cowboy boots in the corner . . . and through the open closet door, on the shelf, I could see a cowboy hat.

In a little while he brought me a complete breakfast on a tray, including fresh orange juice that he had squeezed himself. He sat down on the bed and said, "Good morning, beautiful," and commenced to feed me.

"Where am I," I asked.

"At my place in Sharpstown," he said.

"Is that in the U.S.A.?" And we laughed.

Acting on my inquisitiveness, and with all due respect for this animal's domain, in a well-modulated tone I said, "What are all these guns for?"

Very distinctly, and with a soft touch of abrasiveness in his voice, he said, "Sweetheart, we'll get along just fine, but first you must understand one thing . . . that I operate on a "need to know" basis. Later, I would come to understand the real significance of that kind of operation, and just how it would relate to my life with him.

He said, "Now, there is a time to talk, and a time to eat. This is a time to eat." To my own amazement, I was again, effectively silenced, as he fed me my breakfast in ceremonial fashion. There was an intensity about the operation that held some fascination for me. He did not look at me, only at the plate of food and at my open mouth.

He announced that he must depart for three or four hours, to finish some work at his office. He inquired if I would be all right. (I couldn't imagine that I wouldn't be.) Of course I would. In short order, he carefully arranged the covers, plumped my pillows, and brought me a telephone and one of his company's pagers . . . oh yes, and the Sunday paper. He briefly instructed me on the use of the pager. He told me I could page him if I became ill and needed him, kissed me on the forehead, and in a flash, was gone.

My thoughts returned to that significant sentence, "I operate on a need to know basis." Although there had been a half-smile on his lips, there was no doubt about the seriousness of the message. He left no room for compromise. I wasn't exactly sure what this meant to me, but I don't believe I liked it. The man had grit. No doubt about it. And I liked that. Do you suppose that I might have to make some minor adjustments in my modus operandi? Was this the beginning of the erosion of an independent woman?

It was nine o'clock on Sunday morning and pure terror struck me. My children would be just getting up, and I was not where I was supposed to be . . . in my bed. I telephoned them.

Katie, my eighteen-year-old answered. I was subjected to a barrage of questions, as her voice rose a full octave past her speaking voice. "Mother, where are you? Where did you sleep?" I explained that I had become too ill to travel last night, probably with some deadly virus, and Colonel Becker had suggested that I spend the night in his guest room. I told her that the room was way on the other side of the house. The way I described it, it sounded like it was a block away. I had never stayed out all night. There was a long silence, and then with a degree of urgency in her voice, she said, "Mother, are you sure?" I assured her that I was just fine and that I would see her later on in the evening, after the theater.

The Compost Heap

Toward late afternoon I felt I needed a breath of fresh air, so I slid the glass patio doors open and stepped out. There really wasn't much out there. It was apparent that landscaping was not important to the occupant. There was a barbecue pit, a smoker, and then way back in the rear corner of the lot was a mountain of something. And right on top of it was a large, dented rusty old can with one red rose growing out of the center. This was curious. I would investigate.

I approached the mound . . . and stopped a few feet from the single red rose. A blue jay swooped down and extracted a worm from the heap, and just as quickly, another jay was there scrapping with the first bird over the worm. An instantaneous fierce fight followed. And they were gone. It was then that it came to me. This was a *compost* heap! Merely that and nothing more.

Scenes of my father's funeral floated past in my mind's eye, . . . the lowering of the casket into the ground, the heaps of black dirt and hundreds of red roses. Until I was six years old, I had lived on a farm. Although we later moved from the farm, Daddy always had a compost heap. It was something that was personally his. When I was four or five years old I remember standing out by the compost heap. "What is that, Daddy?" He told me that it was a collection of leaves, clippings and other stuff that was no good to anyone. He said you heap it up into a big pile, and let it "cook" for a long, long time. He said that it turned into something good. He put it on Mama's roses, and it made them big and beautiful. "Sort of like magic?" I said.

"Yes, I believe you could call it magic," he said. I remember thinking what a fine heap of dirt that was, and marveled at how it could make such pretty red roses. From time to time I would visit the compost heap, alone, and just stare at it in amazement. I wondered what was going on in there, to make it do those things. It remained a mystery to me. I would scamper around to the south side of the house, where there seemed to be hundreds of red roses, the prettiest I'd ever seen. There were long moments of reverence, when I gasped at their beauty, and took deep breaths to inhale the fragrance that permeated the air. I would think about the compost heap. The fascination with the process (whatever that was) remained with me for a lifetime.

And here it was in a quiet corner of the world, a beautiful compost heap . . . with one red rose growing in a rusty tin can. I had a quiet communion with this heap of dirt and the red rose. In a way, I was glad to be alone. Things racing in my mind were easier to sort out without the presence of the colonel. Other than my father, I had never known another man with his very own compost heap. There was definitely magic here.

I believe it was at that moment in time that I fell in love, sort of a synergistic situation, I thought.

Every couple of hours, right at the top of the hour, Fritz called to check on my health. I was still in his pajamas and very much in the lounging mode when he arrived around five o'clock. He looked fine. His skin was ruddy and he wore his World War II khakis, and looked much like he was just home from an African safari.

"Sweetheart, you look magnificent," he said, as he swooped me up and swung me around. "Are you hungry?" he asked.

I did feel as if I could eat a bit, so he fixed some soup and a small green salad. Also, he buttered six Ritz crackers and handed three to me. I didn't quite finish the soup, and that did not go unnoticed. He quickly slipped his chair alongside mine, and said, "Now Sweetheart, you must eat all your soup . . . now open." And again, I was mesmerized by the process. "There's a time to talk and a time to eat". . . and so, without a word, and with a steady hand, he fed me all of my soup . . . whether I liked it or not.

An Affair With A Lioness

I sat on the edge of the bed and watched him move methodically about the room. He moved with amazing grace. I was enchanted. Never did he hurry, nor did he dawdle. He moved with a litheness, and without a single wasted motion. He moved with a purpose, with a plan. Yes, I liked him in those khakis. Oh dear, very matter-of-factly, he was removing his shirt, just as if I wasn't there.

When I was about fifteen, there was a period in time when I became enamored with the writings of Rudyard Kipling, who wrote a lot about the jungles, and the animals of the jungles. I became fascinated with the big cats. This man was not unlike one of those cats. Which one? The answer to that question did not come easily to me. I pondered that thought. He was too fair to be a panther, and he had no distinctive markings. No stripes, no spots.

By George, I've got it. He's a lioness . . . even the intensity of his expressions. It really didn't matter that he was not the right gender. He looked like a lioness, most especially, he had a stalking-type walk. In the jungle the lioness is always thinking of where her next meal is coming from, and looking for a piece of meat to kill. I believe this is reflected on her face. They are the hunters for the entire family. How did that arrangement ever evolve? Could it be that the female of the species is the superior hunter?

In time, I would come to know the lioness intimately, and marvel at the striking resemblance of these two enigmatic animals.

Suddenly, my reverie was interrupted with, "A penny for your thoughts?" Instantly I decided that it might be dangerous to let this man inside my head, so early in the game. I looked a long and even look at him, and gave him a supercilious grin. This was probably the beginning of the longtime respect he showed for my privacy, as he didn't repeat the question. He only afforded me a long and even look back.

The bathroom was very close to the bed. He stepped into the bathroom and left the door wide open. I thought, "Heavens, what am I doing here? Things are moving too fast for me." He leaned toward the mirror, lips parted, and thoughtfully examined his face. Slowly, he moved his large hand over his face and jaws. His head moved, like a machine, back and forth, up and down . . . never a second or a millimeter off-course. It was as if he had done this a thousand times. He had. And I found myself caught up in that rhythm.

In the mirror I could see the reflection of his face. I watched in awe, motionless. He set about this process with that same preciseness that seemed to be a way with him. His forearms were thick and sturdy, with lots of curly bronze hair. I was riveted to his reflection.

He took down a straight razor and shaving cream from the cabinet and gently patted and smoothed the cream over his face. I was fascinated. First, I'd never seen a straight razor, and second, it's like he's pretending I'm not here. I was most certainly here, and just about to slip off the edge of the bed. With his big hand, he gripped the razor tightly. In one flowing, careful movement, he began to shave.

My God, why was I obsessed with such passion? I began to feel a little breathless. My face flushed and my eyes became moist. My heart beat hard. I tried to control my extraneous analytic thoughts. I felt a little bit of desperation in this effort to focus, to save the moment. Years later, I would play back this scene in my mind's video. Without a doubt, I count these moments as the most sensuous of many that were to occur on a daily basis.

Lo and behold, the lioness was motionless and looking at me in the mirror with a tinge of determination showing on his face. After a few seconds hesitation, he quietly laid down his razor and dabbed his face with a towel. He said, "I see a beautiful and very respectable looking lady sitting on my bed, and in my pajamas. I'm not complaining. She's a sweetheart, but she looks so serious. I rather like this arrangement with this pretty lady sitting on my bed. She's very quiet. She's thinking. It may be that she is evaluating me. That bothers me."

We were looking at each other, and black magical moments passed between us. I was magnetized. He moved swiftly to resurrect me from the bed, and I was in his arms. His ardent and impetuous kisses and caresses seemed to go on forever. Then with silent consent, we made love.

After the loving, he took me by the hand, and led me into his large closet, where the cowboy hat resided. He said, "Sweetheart, what would you like me to wear to the theater?"

It was a sweet moment, very tender, but I found myself wondering what on earth I was doing in this man's closet. Good grief, one brown suit, two brown suits, three brown suits.

"Don't you have anything but brown suits?" No, he didn't. We had to make do. I tried to perk it up with a tie, but there too, the assortment was dismal. Clearly, this man did not wish to stand out in a crowd. The tie I picked seemed to blend with the brown suit. It looked like little spots of blood on a field of gray ashes in a black pit. I thought, "Wouldn't Freud have liked to have gotten hold of this guy?"

He said, "Sweetheart, would you like to come shopping with me?"

I said, "Would I!"

We spent a delightful evening at the theater. On the way home Fritz asked me if I would like to go see a big old house he owned. It was on Helena Street, and very close. On Helena! Heavens, since 1958 I had been having a continuing love affair with a house on Helena Street. The street was only five blocks long, and this particular house, we discovered, was just a half block from his place. Incredible, I thought.

THE JUNK PILE

Fritz parked in front of his place. Quietly and proudly he admired his own private little junk pile. I couldn't help thinking how close to the earth this man was. Certainly, most men would have hidden this pile of trash, most especially they would have hidden it from a new girlfriend. It said something special to me about this man. It said he was honest and open, like he was saying, "This is me. You can take it or leave it."

It was a big old nineteenth century frame prairie-styled house that was covered with vines. The shrubbery was so overgrown that the house was barely visible. Even so, it had a rather grotesque charm about it. It probably hadn't been painted for twenty-some years. It was a bright night, and in the yard the moon shone on a dozen or so old potties, sinks, piles of cinder blocks, old plantation shutters, stacks of old metal windows, doors, scrap metal and God only knows what . . . of every size and shape. In the side yard there was a clothesline, with men's work clothes hung out to dry. In addition, there were two Volkswagen "bugs," an El Camino, an ancient truck with sideboards, an old washing machine, a deteriorated rowboat and several rusty old car engines.

My God, I'd never before seen such an accumulation of rubbish. I was taken with the affection with which he viewed his treasures. This was a scavenger's delight, with an assortment of items rescued and revered over the years. I suspected that I had a bit of this blood myself. Each item must have a story to tell, and I'll bet he knew just where he had picked up each little piece of trash. I was impressed with the fact that it took such a little piece of trash to bring that look of pride to this man's face. Something basic about his personality was being unabashedly revealed to me, "I am what I am." And that was refreshing.

It was difficult to believe that people were living in this house. Fritz said they were good ol' "Hee Haw" types, a couple in their sixties, and the elderly mother of the woman. They called her "Mama." Fritz said they didn't have a dozen brain cells among them. Jack was the skinny little husband, who was recuperating from a gunshot wound. He worked at a downtown bank as a security guard. A would-be robber knocked him down, took his gun, and shot him in the foot. They were tenants for more than twenty-five years, and probably would still be there if they hadn't become so attached to so many cats. Some four years later, the cat count was twenty-seven. Fritz politely requested that they get rid of all except six cats. How he arrived at that number, I do not know, but I do know that they found this totally unacceptable, and must have viewed it as cruel and unusual punishment. In one week, and without notice, they moved and left the cats for us.

We drove down to the next block, and there was my "Tara". . . a decadent beauty. At least once a year, since 1958, I had driven down here, and just parked and looked and wished it were mine. It was two and a half stories tall, a glorious place with four huge Ionic two-story columns in the front. The architecture was Greek Revival, but the architect had taken some artistic license to slightly depart from the classic style.

One is reminded immediately of a New Orleans townhouse. It was fairly close to the sidewalk, with a lovely bricked courtyard. (Actually, it was not finished and was only bricked on one side.) There was a formal pattern of old boxwoods that were grossly neglected and overgrown to about five feet tall. There was a low brick wall, with a rare nineteenth century acorn-style iron fence on top of the wall. There was a ten to twelve-foot fancy French antique iron gate. The front door was enormous, with a fan-like arched transom above and sparkling cut-and-beveled glass sidelights.

There was a two-story scaffolding in place on the north side of the house. Fritz said it had been there for more than fifteen years.

As we drove slowly away, I identified the house in my own mind. The door was set off-center, on the right side of the house. The major structure was off to the left side. Over the front door, at the second-floor level was a balcony, with balustrades that were repeated on a large third-floor square deck. The roof line, all around, was punctuated with dentils. I thought about the house. And on this evening I commenced to think of it as a minor chord.

We returned to Pemberton Place in West University, to my little brick bungalow with the Mediterranean courtyard and the big southern magnolia tree out front. Fritz parked, and in a tone of voice much like a polite command, turned to me and said, "Now sweetheart, go into the house. Say 'Hello' to your family and grab a few things. I want you to come with me." I hadn't expected this, and was speechless. He kissed me on the forehead, and I did exactly as he asked.

THE BLACK SILK NIGHTGOWN

We returned to the suburbs. We sat in the living room and listened to that sweet clarinet of Pete Fountain, before retiring to bed. Then I donned my lacy long black nightgown and crawled into bed. Fritz said, "What did you put that thing on for?" I ignored his question, and didn't offer to remove it.

He went to the kitchen and returned with several little glasses of Remy Martin. "What are you still doing in that black thing? I thought you were going to take it off," he said.

"No, I didn't say that."

We talked a lot. He talked about growing up in Dallas, and his summer trips to visit his grandparents in San Antonio. In those days it was quite a jaunt. At Christmas time he remembered taking hot bricks on the trip, in order to keep warm. All of his grandparents were born in Germany, and at least two of them were never naturalized. Fritz spoke only German until he was six years old. He was a happy, only child, who was the center of attention on both sides of the family. After Fritz left home, his parents moved from Dallas to San Antonio, where his father's family lived.

His paternal grandparents, and most of his relatives on that side of the family, were very well-educated and socially prominent people. His grandfather was the manager for the opera house, a position he had occupied since it opened, back in the latter part of the nineteenth century. His grandmother was a concert violinist, who was born and reared in Maine, and had given concerts in New York and Boston. Mr. Becker had fetched her from Maine as a bride. Along with her dowry, he had brought her to San Antonio. They had lived in a large house on Broadway, and their property , in the rear, extended all the way to the river. They had many house guests over the years, famous performing artists from around the world. Their lives were filled with parties and many glamorous people were in attendance. His grandmother and aunt were among the founders of the Tuesday Musical Club and the San Antonio Symphony. Fritz said he had the best of both worlds. He said his father's family were aristocrats, and his mother's family were the salt of the earth.

Growing up during the Great Depression was very difficult for Fritz and his family. Actually, their serious financial problems began during the mid-twenties. They lost their home and had to move in with his maternal grandparents. It was difficult keeping body and soul together, and sometimes there was not enough food. His grandfather had a vegetable garden, and his mother and grandmother sold their little bit of jewelry to put food on the table. Their neighborhood grocery store operated an upstairs room where the owners purchased jewelry in exchange for credits in groceries. Like a lot of other people back then, somehow they survived.

It was during this period that the most bruising event of Fritz's young adulthood occurred. He was sixteen and working at a summer job for McKenzie Construction Company. He was instrumental in securing a job for his grandfather at the construction company. Two weeks after he was hired, a dump truck backed over him, instantly killing him. For a long time Fritz felt totally responsible for the death of his grandfather. Later in life he was able to absolve himself of the guilt associated with the accident, but the memory of it stayed with him forever.

We talked until past midnight. He gave me a long and loving caress, and turned out the light.

In the morning I found the black silk nightgown on the floor.

In the days that followed there was no dearth of conversation when we were at home. Like Fritz said, "I go back a long way, Honey, and there's lots to tell."

I drove to my job in Galveston two days a week. Every school day Fritz and I picked up Katie in West University and drove her to The High School for the Performing and Visual Arts. Daily, in the late afternoon, I stopped at my place to organize things. My son, Travis was twenty-three years old and living at home while attending college. My older daughter, Alison, was twenty-five years old and had her own apartment very close by. She had been gone from home for quite some time, since she had gone to The University of Texas in Austin, and had recently graduated. She came by often to visit.

On one of those visits, when both of my daughters were there, the younger one asked that I do her laundry. My older daughter thought this a selfish request. A heated argument ensued. Alison reprimanded Katie severely, pointing out that she was old enough to do her own laundry, and that, "Mother needs to get on with her own life. She's been taking care of you for eighteen years."

Katie did her own laundry and I portioned out the money, made a couple of lists, and left feeling a little bit proud of my children.

The Green-Sculpted Carpeting

I returned late afternoon to the suburbs. Every time I pulled into the driveway, I couldn't believe that I really lived in this unimaginative place. I stepped inside the front door, and again surveyed the interior decor. The piece of furniture which most captured my attention was a huge dark green vinyl chair. It seemed to be the center of life there. It certainly had a personality all of its own. As one sat down in the chair, and reared back, a footrest literally popped up. Later I was told it was called a "Bark-A-Lounger," only it didn't bark. It did utter a long loud squeak when the foot rest popped up. It was a gift from one of his children, as was the green-sculpted carpeting.

Of course, the most outstanding piece was the carved Chinese camphor chest. Elsewhere in the room was a pole lamp with three amber colored glass shades. It reminded me of something I'd once seen at a carnival. Later, Fritz told me that he had purchased it at an IRS auction for three dollars and considered it very functional. All of these things faded into oblivion when we were at home together. They really didn't matter. It did matter that our relationship prospered and permeated the spaces. It seemed that I had attained the highest joy that love could give.

The Gerber Baby

I didn't cook more than a half-dozen meals in those three years that we lived in Sharpstown. Early on, he let me know that his preference was that I stay out of the kitchen. He was a territorial animal, and this was continually revealed to me throughout our lives together.

When we met in the early evenings, he would go directly to the kitchen to start our dinner. Then he would fix a double Manhattan for himself. Usually, he marinated steaks and then grilled them on the patio. Along with the steaks, we had baked potatoes, green beans or corn and a green salad. This was the menu, five out of seven nights. Other times, we had clupsies, which was a recipe from his German grandmother. It was a fried ground meatball mixed with green peppers and onions. The other recipe was a cooked pork roast with mashed potatoes and sauerkraut. It took hours to cook, and smelled up the house. The other diversion from steak was the wonderful authentic enchiladas that he learned how to cook from his San Antonio grandmother. Dessert was always the same. That was Blue Bell Ice cream from Brenham, Texas.

When we sat down to eat he always said the familiar Episcopalian blessing that we said at our house. That made me feel good. Sometimes I needed a gentle reminder of my faith, for God only knows, my conscience gave me enough jabs to remind me that I was a woman "living in sin."

Fritz never wanted to have conversation with dinner. Eating was serious business, and required one's undivided attention. Also, one ate everything on one's plate. At our house dinner was a long drawn out affair, where everyone described in detail what happened that day. So this idea of dinner being a business-like affair seemed alien to me.

When we had steak, he always cut it up into little pieces for me. After that, he would do his little routine of feeding me the steak. It seemed a vicarious pleasure for him. Sometimes he would even open his mouth, (like a mother does when she's feeding her child). Often, after the last bite, he would enthusiastically say, "Good girl." And sometimes I would feel like The Gerber Baby.

Occasionally, when I was alone, I would think about The Gerber Baby, but not for long. I really wanted The Gerber Baby to grow up, but not too quickly. I had read a bit of Freud, but what was this all about? The Gerber Baby thrived, and I was afraid that she would get very fat.

The Agency

Over the years, and from time to time, I would feel the independent woman slipping away, which produced a degree of anxiety inside me.

One day in May I realized that since that first night of our first date, we had spent every night together. There were times when I was alone there that I questioned my good sense. I would wander aimlessly throughout the house, and soak up its strangeness. There were four bedrooms. One of them he used for his office. All of the furniture was government issue, including a desk and five steel filing cabinets. They had locks on all of them. The entire room was functional. Everything, down to the last paper clip, was in its place.

"Heavens, what could possibly be in all those filing cabinets?" I thought. He had presented me with keys to everything, including a tiny brass key that opened these cabinets. Sometimes, when he was in Washington, D.C. on business, or off hunting in Colorado, I would be tempted to take a peek into those files. He had told me I was welcome to go into the files should I need to. Certainly, he wouldn't have given me the keys if there was something secret there. But, I never got past inserting the key in the lock. I would stand there, thinking about what might be in those files, and thinking that this was a very private place. Were there secrets to his past? Goose bumps would erupt on my arms and down my back. My hand would tremble a little, and I would zip the key out of the lock and go away, feeling much like a trespasser.

I remember the first day I went to his office. That was before I had been given the keys. There was a large oak desk with a long desk marker. It had a bird colonel insignia and the Army Engineering Corp's insignia on it. It read "Colonel F.A. Becker." Back in a corner of the desk was a discreet official-looking four-inch-square Lucite memento with a large golden eagle, with its head pointing to the right. It was a familiar-looking logo. I thought, "Where in the world have I seen that damned bird?" It read, "Presented to Fritz A. Becker. in appreciation for twenty-four years of meritorious service."

That was The Central Intelligence Agency's eagle. Indeed it was. I don't believe there has been anything in my background to have prepared me for this. I would visit the library in the morning.

On the wall there was a framed official-looking document that read, "WAR DEPARTMENT CITATION. *Lieutenant Colonel F.A. Becker has distinguished himself by superior, meritorious and faithful performance of services as an officer of the Military Intelligence Service War Department, from 29 January 1942 through 2 September 1945. As Chief of the Southwest Pacific Section and concurrently Executive Officer of the Pacific Branch during most of his service until June 1944, Colonel Becker contributed substantially to the magnitude of accurate intelligence concerning the Pacific Area produced by the MIS during this period and used in the successful planning of the Pacific War. Later as Executive Officer to the Director of Intelligence, Colonel Becker contributed much to the success of the MIS by his skill and effectiveness in implementing the decisions of the Director of Intelligence and particularly by devising an efficient system for coordinating the activities of the components of the Intelligence Group."*

It was dated 29 November 1945. I read it very carefully, and I was impressed.

There was a huge trash can beside the desk. Then, next to that was a piece of equipment I didn't recognize. Later, it was identified to me as a paper shredder.

Sometimes Fritz would mumble in his sleep. Thinking that he was talking to me, I would ask him what he said. He would sit bolt upright and in a somewhat hostile voice say, "DON'T swab me, woman." It was a bit unnerving.

There was something else that made me uneasy, something that I didn't understand. On several occasions Fritz suggested that he teach me how to choke someone to death. I really didn't see why I would need to know this. Fritz explained that I needed to know how to defend myself, and that meant knowing how to kill someone. After some badgering, Fritz won out. I learned just how to choke someone to death.

There were a few other things that bothered me. I didn't like not being welcome in the kitchen. I was not a gourmet cook, but that didn't matter. Also, Fritz insisted on doing all of the grocery shopping. If I selected some produce, he would put it back, and select another specimen. During the process, I was lectured on how to make an intelligent selection.

The first time we returned from grocery shopping, I started to carry in a bag of groceries. "No," Fritz said, "I'll carry all of them in." I asked what I could do to help. He just smiled that infectious smile and said, "Just get in the house, woman and take off your clothes." In all those years, I never carried in another bag of groceries.

Some Sweet Talk

But these things faded into the background. I was totally, desperately and forever in love, and our days and nights were filled with passion.

Every day, all day long, I thought of how I would feel when I saw Fritz again. He would be there waiting with his pinkish smiling face, and he would grab me and swing me around. He would give me a crushing bear hug, and kiss me and kiss me and kiss me.

It was splendid. All through the day, I would lose myself in thoughts of passion. Sometimes he never made it back to the kitchen and we made love before dinner. Sometimes we made love after dinner, too. And sometimes we skipped dinner.

One evening in early June, we attended "Porgy and Bess" at Jones Hall. During intermission we found a secluded corner for some sweet talk. A wave of effervescent desire passed between us, and touched us as we exchanged glances.

After a minute, and out of the blue, and very seriously, Fritz said, "Would you consider marrying me?"

I said, "Yes, I would consider marrying you." And there was no discussion, only a coalescence of our spirits.

Every morning I awakened feeling the seductiveness of our relationship. It was beguiling. It was bewitching. And it sustained me throughout the days.

But sometimes the intensity of our love consumed me, and left me weary. It took its toll. Occasionally it was necessary to take a long afternoon nap, in order to restore my body and soul.

One evening we were in bed, and Fritz had just finished reading aloud "The Little Prince." It was one of my favorite books. He turned out the light and pulled me close to him.

"Sweetheart, there is something I want to discuss with you." It sounded serious. He went on to say, "I would like for us to have a baby. Would you like that?"

I felt as if something had just crashed on top of me. I thought, "Goodness, isn't seven children quite enough?" I didn't say that. I replied, "I don't know. I'm not sure I could handle that. If we did have a child now, I would be in my fifties when the child became a teenager. Also, you've had a vasectomy."

Fritz went on to say that he had read several articles in the paper regarding vasectomy reversal.

I didn't want to say absolutely no, until I had to. I didn't want to offend him.

In the morning he attacked the problem with his usual tenacity, and set up a file marked "VASECTOMY." He made an appointment with a doctor in the medical center. Over the course of the summer, he saw four or five different doctors. He was consumed with his project. It was on his mind from morning until bedtime.

All of the doctors Fritz consulted were of the same opinion; his vasectomy could not be reversed. It had been far too long since the vasectomy had been performed. It had been more than fifteen years. They said the prognosis was poor, and none of them would recommend the surgery. Fritz was extremely disappointed, and I was glad I didn't have to say, "No, at this point in my life, I don't want a baby."

The days passed quickly. Sometimes we did our errands together, and sometimes we parted during the daylight hours. Always we looked forward to when we would meet again, for we knew there would be those magical unending moments when our bodies would be pressed together, and invariably something enigmatic would happen. It was rather like an intellectual celebration of the senses, and it was full of God.

The Beach House

One Friday, just past noon, around six weeks after I had taken up residence with Fritz in the suburbs, he said, "Let's pack up a few things and go to the beach house." Indeed, this was a surprise, for I didn't even know there was a beach house. He had bought it four years before, for an investment, and had only been there twice. It was near Freeport, Texas, at a place called Surfside, on the Gulf of Mexico.

I was jubilant. What a delightful diversion. We packed our swimsuits, one of our dogs, (my wire-haired terrier) and a couple of six-packs of Lone Star. Within an hour we were on the road.

Much of the drive was open, flat farmland. And it gave me a free feeling on this beautiful sunshiny day. I was a woman who was lucky in love, breezing along in a dusty brown Toyota, with only thoughts of loving this man for the rest of my life.

Perhaps I was shoving the single most traumatic event of my entire life deep into my unconscious, but I really didn't give a thought as to where we were going, other than, to Fritz's beach house.

It was not until we turned east, toward the gulf, that I saw a sign that read, "Surfside," that the whole frightful experience re-entered my conscious mind.

It had been fourteen years since my first husband, Tom, had been killed on the way home from a beach outing. The accident happened on this very highway, and on the way home from this very beach.

It had been a Wednesday afternoon, Tom's day off from the clinic where he had been practicing medicine for ten months.

We had spent a wonderful afternoon on the beach, laughing and playing, talking and eating. Tom had said, "Let's do this more often. There's something about the water that brings peace to a man's soul."

After supper the two older children were playing in the surf, when our nine-year-old son was badly bitten by something in the water. Tom examined the painful bite, and believed it to be a snake bite. He treated it by cutting it, in order to express the venom. It was a frightful thing to watch. I threw our belongings into our TR-3, and we were off to the emergency room at Dow Chemical.

It was dusk and we could see the twinkling lights of Dow's refinery as we raced to the emergency room. High anxiety registered on Tom's face. And then in a split second the small sports car, with the side curtains out, hit something and was thrown high in the air. It crashed, upside down on the highway. All of us were thrown from the car. The youngest, four-year-old Katie, was off in the marshes, about fifty feet away. Travis, our nine-year-old son, was the next closest, and Alison, our eleven-year-old, was about five feet from me. I was about fifteen feet from Tom. The front bumper was resting on his leg, and his skull was crushed beyond recognition.

I was quietly frantic, until I uttered a long and blood-curdling scream, after which I went to each child, starting with the youngest, trying to offer some kind of comfort. They were all crying, but appeared to be spared serious injury. Never, in one place, had I seen such a spill of blood. It was everywhere, but much of it came from bad abrasions. Early on, I had told all of the children that it was extremely important that they do not move, but just stay still because they might do further injury to themselves if they moved. Even the four-year-old cooperated. They did exactly as they were told.

Keeping them on the ground served another purpose. I was determined that they not see the grotesque condition of their father's face. For years I lived with that indelible memory.

Darkness came quickly. In retrospect, I don't know how I managed the feat, but after two or three tries I was able to lift the car off Tom's leg.

In about five minutes, a motorist came down the highway and stopped. He went to a nearby grocery store and called for an ambulance.

It was forty-five minutes before the ambulance arrived. During that time, every minute was an eternity, while a million giant mosquitoes sucked our blood.

The people of that little Texas town in Brazoria county were outpouring with love, sympathy, and tons of food. They had loved their doctor who made house calls. In ten months he had made a reputation for himself. Not only did he make house calls, he carried a green fishing tackle box instead of a black bag. That was because it was easily organized.

As I glanced across at Fritz I couldn't help but being reminded of the many similarities that existed between the two men. The were both brilliant, and highly organized. And although it had never been directed at me, they both had a touch of temper. Both had German grandparents, and both had at least two great-grandparents who were Irish. They were both a little better than six feet tall with the same pinkish complexion and blue-gray eyes. One was graduated in electrical engineering and the other had studied electrical engineering for two years and then changed to medicine. He later had become a physician. Both of them could fix any broken mechanical thing, and that was very handy. More importantly, they were both self-made men.

Early on I had told Fritz a bit about the accident, but certainly he didn't know just where it had occurred, nor did he know any of the details. It was not that I was keeping any of this from him, it was just that there had never been a right time to reveal the entire story.

Fritz looked across at me and said, "Honey, are you all right? You look as if you might be a little sick."

I assured him that I was all right, but if the truth were known, I didn't feel so hot.

As we drove the remaining five or six miles, I lay my head back and closed my eyes. I didn't want to see the place on the highway where the accident had occurred.

Fritz said, "Wake up, Sweetheart. We're almost to the beach house."

I opened my eyes to see the big bridge that spanned the Intracoastal Canal . . . and there was the Gulf of Mexico. As we crossed the bridge, I realized that our last picnic on the beach had taken place just off to the left, after crossing the bridge. Oh God, we turned left and drove up the beach about a block. And there was the spot where we had that last picnic, directly in front of Fritz's beach house. I was dumfounded. I took a deep breath, and wanted to run away.

The house was right on the beach. It was a two bedroom cottage, up on stilts, with a nice front porch.

Weakly, I got out of the car, and Willie, the terrier, high-tailed it down to the water, and I went after him. Fritz went up to the house. I was hoping to recover from the shock of the situation, but things worsened before they got better.

I sat down close to the water's edge, and took some deep breaths, while Willie frolicked in the surf.

Fritz was calling, “Liz, come up here. The house has been broken into and vandalized.”

I called the dog from the water and started toward the house. There were huge sand dunes between the water and the house. This made walking slow and difficult. I was hot, and beginning to feel weak. That last picnic here, and the aftermath of that hideous accident flashed in my mind’s eye, and something in my head went round and round, as I collapsed on the dunes.

When I regained consciousness, I awakened with my head in Fritz’s lap, and cold wet towels on my head.

“Sweetheart, what happened? Did the heat get you?” Fritz said.

“It seems that it did,” I said. Someday I would tell him, but I knew that right now, inside me, the stamina simply didn’t exist to get me through the horrible account of the accident. I smiled a wan smile as he slowly bent down and kissed me delicately on the lips. Communicated in that kiss, was a message, a message of knowing that he knew I felt pain. And in one direct sentence he said, “Sweetheart, I know that you have suffered, and I wish more than anything, there was something I could do about that.”

TYLER, TEXAS AND THE LOS ANGELES ROSE

Toward the end of June, we took a motor trip to Tyler, Texas, where one of Fritz's sons lived with his family. It would be Father's Day, and his oldest daughter, Brenda, was coming to visit. She lived in Los Angeles. He said he really didn't want to go, but felt he had to. I thought that a strange way of feeling.

Fritz had said very little about his children since I'd known him. After a while I could see that he really avoided any contact with them. I thought that was unusual. I had met all of his children, except the daughter from California, whom he had only mentioned in passing.

On the trip to Tyler, he said, "Brenda is beautiful, skinny, but beautiful . . . not the kind of woman a man would want. She's smart, but very self-centered and selfish." He went on to say how he felt sorry for her husband, that he would hate to have to be married to her, and finished it off with, "She's a bitch." And that was that. I was startled by this not-too-complimentary description of his daughter.

When we met for the first time, Brenda embraced her father with a big hug, while she afforded me a chilly "Hello." All of us visited for about forty-five minutes. Then Brenda suggested the two of us walk outside to visit. Once outside, she looked at me with wild dancing eyes, and in an agitated voice said, "What are your plans for my father?"

I was shocked. I told her I didn't really know exactly what she meant, but we were living together and enjoying ourselves. She asked if I was planning to marry him. I replied that her father had asked, but for now, we certainly had no such immediate plans. She snapped, "That's not what Dad told me."

I said, "Well, you can be sure that if and when we do marry, you'll be notified."

I went inside and reported the nasty encounter to Fritz. He was furious, and wanted to "dress her down." Also, he wanted to leave for home immediately. I discouraged that. He said, "That bitch. My Goddamned children just won't leave me alone... about you."

And so we stayed, against Fritz's protestations, for the long two days. It was very strained. On the way back to Houston the next evening he said, "We never should have come up here, and remind me to stay away from my children, and I hope that bitch stays in California."

And we were glad to be back to the house with the green-sculpted carpeting, and glad to be back in each others arms, and glad to be back on our king-sized bed.

"Lavender's Blue, Dilly Dilly"

The summer of 1976 brought us closer together. We spent a lot of time at the beach house. It had been badly vandalized. There were almost one hundred window panes broken out. Broken glass covered the entire house. Some of the furniture, and some of the dishes were also broken. And if that weren't bad enough, there were multiple water pipes leaking in and under the house. Being the worker that he was, Fritz was happy to be off to the hardware store to purchase what he needed to make the necessary repairs. I assisted with the repairs, along with redoing the interior of the house. Between the two of us, we managed to scrounge up some pretty nifty furniture. I bought some red-and-white plaid curtains for the kitchen and some white ruffled cottage curtains for the rest of the house.

When I worked in Galveston, I would drive down to the beach house to meet Fritz. It was a forty-five-minute drive along the beach. There was very little traffic, and I would set the radio on the classical music station, turn up the volume, and enjoy the drive.

One day, I stopped at an antique shop in Galveston, and bought an old English Axminister rug for the beach house. I was delighted, and Fritz was pleased.

By the first part of August everything was repaired, and again, the beach house was livable. We sat on the front porch drinking our coffee and watching the sun rise, and Fritz hugged me hard and said, "Sweetheart, this is our very first house that we've done together." And I felt content. We finished our coffee, and then walked hand in hand up the beach, gathering shells along the way.

When the moon was full, we almost always took a long walk on the beach. Actually, most nights we walked on the beach. It was a serene and beautiful way to end the day.

We spent many days and many nights at the beach house during July and August, whiling away the days and loving away the nights. It was pure joy.

One day, in Houston, we passed a Mercedes dealership. We stopped to look. We bought a beautiful black diesel sedan, with leather upholstery. This became the car in which we did most of our traveling, and the car Fritz referred to as "Liz's car." My Volvo station wagon became the beach car, and the car we used to haul things, and God knows, we did plenty of that.

In mid-August I fell ill with a headache. From the beginning I knew that this was not just an everyday, run-of-the mill headache. I probably had only had a dozen headaches in my entire life. It persisted, increasing in intensity, for five or six days. Finally, I visited my internist, who diagnosed it as occipital neuritis and referred me for x-rays. I chose the radiologist that my husband had trained under at Baylor College of Medicine.

By this time, I was very sick, with a severe headache in the back of my head. I was nauseated and had begun to lose weight. I was in dire need of sleep. I couldn't lay my head down to sleep, so I had to try to sleep sitting up. When I tried to lay my head down to sleep, it felt as if it were exploding. I was frightened, for I knew that something was very wrong.

During this time I had the most wonderful and attentive nurse. He tended me, oh-so-carefully and kept a twenty-four-hour vigil. All night long he strummed his uke and sang songs to me . . ."Lavender's blue, dilly dilly," "Ain't she sweet? See her coming down the street," "Easter Parade," "Honey," and many more.

Thinking that I might have a brain tumor, my mind went crazy with morbid thoughts surrounding my demise. My doctor suggested that I be hospitalized, but Fritz convinced him that he knew just how to care for me.

My friend, the radiologist, found that I indeed did not have a brain tumor. (I certainly did a lot of praying.) What I did have was encephalitis. I was ill for several months, and during that time there was a new dedication of my love for Fritz. He left the house only to shop for food and medicine. He was totally consumed with the chore of restoring me to good health. Sometimes I would become lost in reverie as I observed his meticulous involvement in caring for me. Indeed, I was in awe of the attentiveness of the lioness. Besides the music he provided, he read the newspaper aloud to me every day, and read a number of books to me.

After a month or so, when I began to feel better, we planned an extensive motor trip up the east coast. Our destination was Bar Harbor, Maine. Our plans included a stop in New Orleans, for some jazz, and a long drive through the Great Smokey Mountains, then on up through the Blue Ridge Mountains of Virginia. We would visit some of our friends and family in the Washington, D.C. area. We decided always to take the scenic routes, and never to make reservations. We marked the positions of all of our friends and relatives on a map. Then we scratched two-thirds of those.

With love, tenderness, and a lot of attention from Fritz, my recovery was accelerated. By mid-October, we were ready to set out on our loosely-planned journey.

A Bat Out of Hell

The evening before we left, Fritz came home with a dozen ears of fresh corn-on-the-cob. I wondered how on earth we would eat that much corn before we left. He said they were a dozen ears for a dollar, and we would have no problem if we just made a meal of the corn. He and his mother used to do that often. He was right. We had no problem finishing the corn, and we retired early for a good nights sleep before the start of our trip in the morning.

After breakfast I found a precious little step ladder in the closet, with a note attached. It read, "Sweetheart, I hope this makes life a little easier for you. Love, Fritz." I was touched.

Our black Mercedes was packed, and all of the necessities for travel were assembled. Our cash was stashed, along with our atlas and maps. The day before leaving, my children gathered with us and we said our good-byes, along with their prayers. From the beginning they said, "Mr. Becker, you drive just like Mother . . . like a bat out of hell." Of course, neither of us understood what they were talking about.

We headed out east, into the sunrise, toward Beaumont. As we glanced at each other, a look of joy and anticipation registered on our faces.

After we crossed into Louisiana, we stopped for a late lunch of some wonderful Cajun food. Then we headed up along the Mississippi river towards Vicksburg. It was a Confederate stronghold, and the town is high upon a bluff on the Mississippi River. I had a special interest in Vicksburg. It was my great-great-great grandfather, Reverend Newet Vick, who founded the town. We spent several days in Vicksburg at a nineteenth century inn. The furniture was all of the period, and we slept in a Prudent Mallard rosewood full tester bed. All of our meals were served in the formal dining room, with antique china and sterling.

We left Vicksburg and headed down along the Mississippi River to New Orleans, where we stayed at an old hotel in the French Quarter. It had the most beautiful antique French ironwork. We arrived in the late afternoon, and after a stroll down Bourbon Street, Fritz found the friendly pub at the hotel. We had a few drinks with a couple from Oklahoma, and then had dinner with them in the hotel dining room.

We stayed in New Orleans for four days, antiquing, eating quite a lot of French food, and listening to Dixieland jazz until early in the mornings.

The next three days we spent traveling up through Mississippi, Alabama and Tennessee, and on through the Great Smokey Mountains.

The weather was bright and chilly and the mountains were glorious. There was a rushing mountain stream that followed the winding road for many miles. We stopped and spent some time walking along the stream, while we listened to the sound of the water.

Several rafts, with boisterous college-aged kids, came rushing by. We had a discussion about renting a raft, but Fritz thought he'd rather not. He did say that he'd go along for the ride! I gave up that idea.

The changing colors of the leaves were spectacular and lifted our spirits. We wanted to stay in the mountains, and we did. We found a wonderful little log cabin inn with a big stone fireplace. There was a small, cozy dining room where we could look out into the woods and see a mountain stream.

We settled in and were so comfortable we must have stayed at least a week. Every day we spent a lot of time wandering in the woods and walking along the stream. We sat by the fire for hours, talking and reading aloud. We read "Daphnis and Chloe" which was illustrated by Marc Chagall. The glow from the fire afforded me a warmth that was in tune with my feelings of comfort and security. As I glanced across at Fritz, flickering firelight played on his rugged face, and I thought that I wanted time to stop moving, because certainly this is the way I wanted to feel for the rest of my life. Yet, at the same time, I felt a certain fragility of the moment, like there would likely be times in the future when I would have to fight to keep these feelings alive. Occasionally, we visited with the other guests. I also remember eating a lot of good catfish and sipping Remy Martin by the fire after supper.

THE PERILOUS PICNIC

One crisp sunny morning we decided to move on. We traveled in a northeasterly direction, following the Appalachian chain. Mid afternoon we stopped at a little grocery and bought the makings for sandwiches and some beer. We found a perfect picnic spot on a high plateau that overlooked the valley. I guess one would say we were on top of the mountain. We spread out our blanket and put together the ham and cheese sandwiches. Fritz popped open a couple of beers and said, "Sweetheart, we're in high cotton," and he grabbed me and kissed me and swung me around.

There hadn't been a single car that passed by, until we heard the unmistakable sound of a Chevy engine coming down the road. It was a beat-up blue pickup and it pulled right in alongside us. We were just a little bit startled. We surveyed the intruders as they jumped from their truck. They were a couple of long-haired, unkempt-looking punks in dirty bluejeans and trashed-out Reeboks. One wore a leather jacket, and the other a Redskins sweatshirt. One was short, blond and stocky, and the other, tall, thin, and with dirty brown unruly hair. I guessed them to be in their mid-twenties. Fritz was halfway on his feet when the short one pushed him on the shoulder very aggressively and said, "Sit down, Tex... mind if we sit down?" Fritz said, "No, have a seat. I'm Fritz Becker from Houston, Texas. Sit down."

Then the short one said, "Tex, do you suppose you could fix me a sandwich? And how about a beer?"

Fritz said, "Sure, we've got plenty of food and beer."

The skinny one did most of the talking. There was a pause in the conversation, and then he said, "Tex, I sure do like them cowboy boots."

I quickly made them sandwiches, and Fritz gave them beers. At the same time, I was trying to get some kind of reading from Fritz as to what might be going on here. To me, these guys just didn't look as if they could be trusted. I was frightened, but Fritz just looked as if it was just one happy little picnic, while I was thinking that it would certainly be a beautiful place to die.

They scarfed up the sandwiches and helped themselves to the two remaining beers. Then they struck up a conversation with Fritz about Texas, and horses and cowboys. Their interest seemed genuine. They spoke a dialect I couldn't quite identify, but I made a guess that they were from deep in the hills of Appalachia.

I thought about our cash reserve, and felt reasonably safe, since it rested next to my heart. Also, my jewelry was hidden in a little velvet pouch in the spare tire well. They finished their beer, and tossed the cans into the weeds beside the trash can.

Suddenly, the tall skinny one stood up and said, "O.K. Cowboy, give me your wallet and your Rolex watch." GOD, he was holding a shiny steel-blue pistol to Fritz's head. I was praying that Fritz would not be a stubborn German, and that he would cooperate. He seemed to be thinking it over, and then the skinny one kicked him in the rear and hollered, "Tex, I said gimme your wallet and your watch, NOW."

Fritz quickly complied. Then they emptied out my purse and between the two of us we figure they got less than fifty dollars in cash. We sat motionless, as they took out toward their truck. Then the skinny one turned around and walked back toward Fritz. He said, "Tex, I think I want them cowboy boots."

Fritz afforded him a long and mean look, and then tossed the boots onto the ground. The skinny one picked them up and said, "Thanks, Tex," and they were gone.

"Let's get the hell out of here," Fritz hollered, as he jumped in the car. I shoved the contents of my purse back into my purse, grabbed our blanket, and we were on our way.

Several miles down the road we came to a sign that read, "Johnson City," which was in the direction of the Interstate. In Johnson City, we found the police station and reported our confrontation with the bandits. That was the last we ever heard of that.

YANKEE STADIUM

For now, we'd had enough of the mountains, so we got on the Interstate, and headed toward Washington, D.C. I had a number of friends and family in the D.C. area and the surrounding suburban Maryland and Virginia areas. We spent about five days there.

We were, however, eager to be on the road again, and happy to be alone in our black Mercedes cocoon. I leaned over and gave Fritz a couple of kisses on the side of his face. Instead of going straight to the Beltway, he turned into Rock Creek Park, and pulled into a playground area alongside the creek.

He grabbed me at the top of both arms and said, "Sweetheart, I haven't told you for a few days, but you're beautiful . . . and I love you more than you know." And he kissed me and kissed me and kissed me, all over my face.

We left the park, picked up the Beltway, and headed north on Route 1 toward New England. We passed through Maryland, Delaware, New Jersey, Pennsylvania, and then we found ourselves in downtown Manhattan at rush hour. It had been our intention to bypass the city, but somehow we missed our turn. We were hopelessly lost, and it was dusk. Then it was dark. We passed the blue-lighted Yankee Stadium sign five times. Finally, we found our way to The Plaza Hotel. We checked in, sorted ourselves out, and had a marvelous dinner on Palm Court.

In the morning we had breakfast sent up to our room. We lingered over our coffee, and then went back to bed.

During the next three weeks we spent a lot of time in Connecticut, along Long Island Sound. Then we traveled on to the Boston area. We spent about five days on the north shore, and visited Salem, Marblehead, Rockport and Olde Newbury, the town my mother's family helped found in 1635.

We drove along the coast, through New Hampshire, and all along the Maine coast up to Bar Harbor.

It was the end of November when we arrived in Bar Harbor. It had gotten very cold and there was something in the air. It was snow, and we were shivering. Not only was it snowing, it was twenty-five degrees, and with a forecast of ten degrees for the next day.

The penetrating cold cut short our stay, and we took out for Texas. We yearned for the Texas sun, and we missed our dogs. We spent very little time in any one place on the trip home. When we arrived in Houston on December 15, the sun was shining and it was seventy-five degrees. We were rather glad to be home, glad to romp with our dogs, and glad to be back on our king-sized bed, and we celebrated.

Christmas Cheer

During Christmas of 1976, I came to know Fritz's family just a little bit better. His son hosted a family party, to which I was not invited. Fritz refused to go without me, so I agreed to join him. Everyone in attendance received a gift except me. Fritz silently seethed with anger. We left early, and just out the door Fritz said, "I don't want to ever come here again. I've got a bunch of reprobates for children."

During 1977 our extravagant and passionate love affair flourished. Often I thought of how lucky I was, and the difference this man had made in my life. He told me how I had made his life complete, and how he felt like he was seventeen again. Still, we hurried home in the afternoons, to touch each other again . . . for what always seemed to be the very first time.

From time to time we visited the Greek Revival house on Helena Street. During one of these visits, Fritz said to me, "Sweetheart, I'm going to buy this house for you . . . and I'm going to fix it up so that it's the most beautiful house in Houston."

I was ecstatic, and we hugged and danced on the sidewalk. Again, I was reminded, that we were both dreamers.

The Helena Street house had a large iron gate and a huge chain wrapped around it with a padlock. There was no way we could get to the door to knock. We went by the house every day for several months. The chain was always on the gate.

Finally, after a couple of months, we noticed the gate was unlocked. As we approached the door, the sheer curtain moved. We heard a radio playing, but we could not get anyone to answer the door. Later, neighbors told us that the man living there was a recluse.

During March, April and May, we spent a lot of time at the beach house. The beach was deserted and we shared it with the gulls. Indeed, it was peaceful. Always, when there was a storm brewing in the gulf, or a hurricane, we packed up and scampered to the gulf. We were drawn to the howling wind, the blowing rain, and the turbulent surf pounding against the dunes in front of the house. There was no television or telephone, only a radio. We listened to a lot of classical music. Fritz was beginning to enjoy my music, and most especially opera. He would say, "Sweetheart, it's almost as good as jazz. How is it that I've lived this long and I'm just discovering opera?"

Ever since we first met, Fritz and I had regularly visited his eighty-four-year-old mother, who was bedridden and in a nursing home. She had severe arteriosclerosis with senile dementia. She did not recognize Fritz and said only two things, "I'm hungry," and "I want to go home." It was quite pitiful, but I was touched with the sweetness and tenderness with which Fritz handled his mother. He spent most of the visit petting her, and stroking her brow.

After one of these visits, we walked to the car in silence. We got in, and Fritz turned, looked straight at me and very seriously said, "If I ever get like my mother, I want you to put me in a nursing home. Do you understand?" There was a long silence and I said, "No, I couldn't do that."

In the fall we spent most of October in the Texas hill country. We stayed at a small inn on the Guadalupe River. We hiked in the hills, rode horses, and laughed as we walked along the Guadalupe.

When we returned to Houston we went straight to the Greek Revival house on Helena Street. Lo and behold, the padlock was gone. The owner came to the door, and we introduced ourselves. He invited us in. We informed him of our interest in buying his house. He told us he would think it over, and be back in touch. We were happy and hopeful, and as we departed, we imagined ourselves already living there.

The year 1978 did not begin well. During the first week, Fritz became very ill with severe chest pains. Against his protestations, I rushed him to the emergency room. He was immediately hospitalized with severe angina. He would have to wait three weeks to get on Dr. Denton Cooley's surgery schedule, for a triple bypass operation and the installation of a pacemaker. I can only say that I was scared to death.

We were able to get a room with two beds, so for the next six weeks I lived at St. Luke's Hospital in the medical center in Houston. For Fritz's benefit, I took on a very courageous attitude. It was all superficial. I was clearly distressed, and there was a little tremor deep inside me. I thought, "What if ? . . . What if ?" Suddenly, I realized the distinct possibility existed that I might have to live my life without him. The thought was unthinkable, and quickly I changed the direction of my thinking.

Immediately, I notified all of Fritz's children that he was in the hospital, and the date of his surgery. None of them came to visit, even though four of them lived in Houston.

The Sunday afternoon before surgery, my three children, a close friend named Dorothy, two of Fritz's former secretaries and I spent the afternoon with him in his hospital room. I learned that all of my children had donated blood for Fritz. This surprised and pleased him. In the two years they had known him, they had become unexpectedly close. There wasn't too much he wouldn't do for them. As a matter of fact, he just plain spoiled them.

Myra and Carolyn had been Fritz's secretaries at the C.I.A. Carolyn said, "Liz, Fritz's children are conspicuous by their absence, but I would have been surprised if they had been here." It was unbelievable that not one of his seven children was there to wish him well. Fritz was in very good spirits, and seemed to be enjoying the attention. There was no mention of his children by him. He had a unique way of compartmentalizing his life and could erase their existence at will.

The surgery was a total success. That evening, during the last five minutes of visiting hours, one of Fritz's sons came rushing in to visit him in intensive care.

After three weeks Fritz was discharged and we returned to his place. His recovery was truly remarkable. We started a program of walking every day and our diet was radically changed. We now ate a low-fat diet with very little meat, a lot of fruits and vegetables, and sometimes a little bit of ice cream.

By May, Fritz was back to his old on-the-go self. He went to his office part of the day, bowled in two bowling leagues, attended a Rotary lunch each week, and still found quite a lot of time to spend with me.

In mid May, Fritz's mother-in-law from his first marriage, who had always been a royal thorn in his side, died. His daughter, Brenda, from Los Angeles, attended the funeral with Fritz. Several days after the funeral, she gave an estate sale of her newly inherited belongings. Fritz returned after the sale looking mad and mean. He had asked Brenda if he could use her late grandmother's wheelchair for his mother, and when she passed on, he would sell it and send the money along to her. She was very short with him and refused to consider that arrangement. She said, "No Dad, I want the money now." He wrote her a check for the wheelchair.

Fritz was smoking mad, and said, "Sweetheart, is there something special that I can do for you?"

I said, "Yes, take me out for some Chinese food for dinner." During dinner, Fritz said, "Not one of my children takes after me, and I hope that damned woman goes back to California, and stays there."

Early one evening, Fritz burst through the door and picked me up, put me down, and with a grin on his face said, "Are you ready to move downtown?" He had just talked to the gentleman who owned the house on Helena and had made an appointment to write a contract in the morning. This was extraordinary. I was going to have the house that I had fallen in love with twenty years ago.

By mid June we were the very proud owners of a great house that needed a ton of work. Actually, by our standards, it was not habitable. I am sure that the wretched condition of the house was what Fritz found most attractive. Here he had found a project that could provide him work for the rest of his life. I believe this pleased him.

We found a contractor who was agreeable to Fritz working on the job with him. Work began immediately. It took three weeks to gut the house and carry away the rubbish. Fritz spent most of his days working with the contractor and I spent my time at the Decorative Center and shopping with Fritz for equipment and supplies.

During August, Fritz's eighty-six-year-old mother died. After the funeral, that night in bed, Fritz looked straight at me and said, "Sweetheart, if I should lose my mind, like my mother, I don't want to live. You're a very smart woman, and if you don't know how to carry out my wishes, then you make it your business to find out."

I was speechless and just lay in silence. Then he kissed me good-night, and I lay in the darkness wondering just how I would do that, should it become necessary.

We worked on the house from dawn until dusk, through the summer and into the fall. There was neither heating nor air conditioning, and no kitchen or bathroom. Working in the heat of the summer was difficult. In the fall Fritz began to completely rewire all three floors of the house. Except for two weeks in November, when Fritz went hunting in Colorado, he worked all through the winter. It was very cold, around forty degrees, and it was colder inside the house than outside. Fritz wore his warm hunting clothes and a stocking cap that I had knitted for him. Sometimes I would help him pull wires. I couldn't pry him away from his work, even for lunch. Every day I made sandwiches and brought him a thermos of hot coffee. I count those intimate lunches among the most romantic that I remember.

In February of 1979 we made the decision that it was necessary to move into the house, even without a kitchen or bathroom. Because the house was vacant, it was an attraction for burglars, and we were broken into five times. We lost a lot of antique fixtures and some very expensive power tools.

Fritz sold his house in the suburbs and on April 30th we moved into our beautiful house that still was without any of the amenities for normal living. Even without all the comforts, living there was pure joy. Fritz had installed a huge skylight on the third floor, so we made our bed on the floor under the skylight. From the third floor deck we had a spectacular view of downtown Houston. The upstairs of the big old duplex Fritz owned, down the street, was vacant. We were able to use the bathroom and kitchen. That was a blessing.

One bright and balmy night, around the nineteenth of May we were on the third floor deck, watching the moon rise. Fritz turned to me and said, "Sweetheart, almost three years ago

I asked if you would consider marrying me. So what has come out of your considerations?"

Four days later, we would be married.

A WEDDING AND THE MARIACHIS

We were married Memorial Day weekend, on a Friday afternoon, the 25th of May, 1979 at Palmer Memorial Episcopal Church on Main Street in Houston. It was a small intimate wedding with only about thirty guests. Fritz wore his navy pinstripe suit, with a red carnation in his lapel. I wore an Oscar de la Renta silk organza, hand-blocked floral print long dress. It was red, white, navy and purple with long purple streamers from the waist. I wore my hair in a French twist, with fresh flowers, and purple streamers down the back. During the wedding ceremony, when the priest asked Fritz to kiss me, a huge thumb gouged me in the armpit and ripped a five-inch-tear in my dress. Fritz whispered in my ear, "Sweetheart, we're in high cotton."

During the three years that Fritz and I were together before our marriage, his children did everything humanly possible to sever our alliance. The harder they tried, the more angry and determined Fritz was to preserve our relationship. Actually, only a few good feelings existed between Fritz and his children, and now I could see that they were demolishing the little bit that was left. He would only say, "I want those kids out of my life." We grew closer.

Five of his children reluctantly attended our wedding, and they really didn't look especially happy to be there.

Our reception was on the church courtyard. The food was catered by our friend, Dorothy, and we had four cases of Spanish Codorniu. Everyone had a delightful time, except for Fritz's children. There were no "congratulations" or "best wishes" from them. The reception lasted for five hours. I overheard Fritz telling his best man, "I always said I'd *never* marry a stuck-up Yankee bitch."

Because we'd just gotten married, we saw no reason why we shouldn't spend the night in our attic room. As we approached our house, we heard music. It was mariachi music. Across the street from our place was a big house, where a large Mexican family lived. There were lots of people in the yard, and they were singing and dancing to the mariachi music. There were several guitars, a violin, an accordion and some castanets. Several of the men who spoke English invited us to join them. They were cooking barbecue outside, and when they learned that we'd just been married, they played mariachi wedding music. They invited us for dinner. Their hospitality was enormous. They threw some more ribs on the grill, sent out for some more beer, and returned with a bouquet of flowers for me. When they learned that Fritz was a musician, they persuaded him to go across the street for his ukulele. He had a great time playing with them. The music was festive and joyful. The supper was delicious, and we danced until past midnight.

It was a great homecoming. In the years to come, weather permitting, almost every weekend we joined our neighbors for barbecue, beer and mariachi music.

The summer was long, and hot as blue hell, ninety to one hundred degrees, plus. We purchased a fan for the attic, where we were still sleeping.

By October, our custom-made kitchen had been delivered, and by December the kitchen had been installed. We also had hot and cold running water and a functioning bathroom. Everything was coming together, but there was still a lot of work to be done.

This was the first Christmas in our house, and even though we had no furniture in our living and dining rooms (only power tools, table saw and lumber), we were ecstatic. We decorated a Christmas tree and Fritz serenaded me on his ukulele with "Jingle Bells" and "Cielito Lindo," and "Deck the Halls." All of my senses seemed to overcome me, and I thought I would die of love.

Although Fritz did not welcome their visit, (and in fact clearly said he wished they would stay away), his son and family did come for their annual forty-five-minute visit. His daughter in California sent us a honey-baked ham. We took half of it to an elderly poor neighbor, where it was enthusiastically received.

Before Christmas we took a three-week break from our work on the house. It was such fun . . . Christmas shopping at Neiman-Marcus and Saks Fifth Avenue. There were crowds of scurrying people, Christmas bells tolling, and Christmas music, and we found ourselves singing along to "Joy to the World."

From January to August we worked on putting down hardwood flooring, finishing it, shopping for and installing chandeliers and lighting fixtures, and finishing the baseboards and crown moldings.

Early in the year I hired a part time housekeeper, named Pat. She was a young Afro-American who was jovial and pleasant to have around. Fritz didn't really want a maid. It took a while for me to figure out that he only wanted the two of us in the house. He said, "We don't need anyone here except you and me. We don't need a maid. We can do everything ourselves. What do we need a maid for?"

In August there appeared a tropical depression in the gulf. Quickly, we packed up and took off for the beach house. On the second day the tropical depression was upgraded to a hurricane. By the third day we heard on the radio that hurricane Allen was expected to hit the Gulf coast of Texas. The winds picked up and the tides rose. They announced on the radio that everyone living in our area should evacuate. We thought certainly, that was just for the faint-at-heart and scaredy-cats.

On the morning of the fourth day we stepped out on the porch on the storm's side and facing the Gulf. The strong wind just about blew us down. The sky was dark and the surf was higher than I'd ever seen it. The wind was so loud I couldn't hear Fritz, even when he hollered. It was quite a storm, and we were intoxicated by it.

Fritz fixed a good breakfast. After eating we got into our big four wheel drive truck and drove along the beach, until we got into some high water and had to retreat. The storm was exciting, but it was also ominous.

Shortly after we returned from our excursion, there came a knock on our door. It was a man from the sheriff's department strongly urging us to leave the area. He told us the hurricane was expected to come ashore tomorrow and that we were in a very dangerous position.

After he left, we discussed the situation. I told Fritz how my first husband and I had stayed in the town of Sweeney, Texas, when most people had evacuated, during hurricane Carla in 1961. We took a two-hour expedition in our TR-3, out into the eye of the hurricane. It was something I wouldn't have missed for anything.

Regardless of our visitor, I think we already knew that we would ride out the hurricane. After all, wasn't this what we had come for?

We spent the afternoon reading aloud from Edgar Allen Poe's work. Also, we took an energetic, invigorating walk on the beach. Our plans were to walk to the pier that was a mile away, but walking became difficult due to the strong wind, so after a half-hour or so, we abandoned our plan.

We had an early supper of my most favorite hot dogs, after which we spent a few minutes on the porch checking out the wind velocity. Indeed, the wind was quite a bit stronger, and not wanting to get blown away, we hurried back inside.

We retired to bed early, and Fritz brought us little glasses of Remy Martin. The wind howled around the cabin. It was a perfect night for reading Poe's, "The Raven." After the bedtime story, and checking out the weather report, we turned out the light. The hurricane was expected to come ashore tomorrow, between Freeport and Brownsville.

I wasn't sure how long we had been asleep, but there came an urgent and loud banging at the door. Fritz grabbed his gun, went to the door and asked who was there. It was the sheriff. Fritz put his gun away and invited him in. He gave us a short lecture on why we must leave immediately, and ordered us to vacate. He said the tide could rise high enough that the houses could flood, along with the road to the bridge over the Intracoastal Canal. That would mean we could not escape. The bridge road was the only way out. He said we were the only people left in the area.

He left quickly, but only after we gave him our assurance that we would leave immediately. We packed our things, grabbed our dog, and were gone within ten minutes.

We drove home in the wind and the rain and arrived in Houston around two o'clock in the morning. The next day hurricane Allen came ashore at Brownsville, Texas.

Certainly, we were disappointed that we were ordered to leave the beach house, but we were also glad to be home and back to work on our house. During October we concentrated our work on the gardens outside. In November and December we spent quite a lot of time just sitting by the fire. Fritz very quickly became attached to the fireplace. He loved chopping the wood, stoking the fire and cleaning up and hauling out the ashes. He had installed the fireplace, including the Louis XVI marble mantel. We put a small round table in front of the fire, and took most of our meals there in winter.

Bad Blood

My most outstanding memory of Christmas 1980 is the gift we received from Fritz's daughter in California. It was one-half of a honey-baked ham! The year before she sent a whole ham and we gave half of it to an elderly poor neighbor. Fritz picked up the one-half ham and stomped out, banging the door behind him. For some reason, I thought the whole episode quite amusing. Fritz did not. He returned, very angry with his daughter and said, "Tell Brenda that we gave the ham to the Petersons again. You know, not one of my children looks like me, or acts like me. All of them have that bad Carter blood coursing through their veins."

During 1981 we continued work on our house. We still had not finished shopping for lighting fixtures, so we spent a great deal of time looking for antique chandeliers and fixtures. We traveled to Dallas, Fort Worth, San Antonio, New Orleans and Natchez.

In February I bought a large wooden easel, and since we no longer slept in the attic, I set up my painting studio there. My first work was a large red poppy, about four by four feet. It rather characterized my life during that period. It a was a big, warm, friendly and happy flower. Fritz loved it, and used to say, "You and your poppy make me feel good." It now hangs in my stairwell.

LOTTIE MAE'S SECRET

In the spring I remember one particular trip to the beach house. Sometimes we stopped to visit Fritz's blind and severely retarded son who lived in the country with an older Afro-American couple. Lottie Mae had been the full time housekeeper for about fifteen years when he was married to his first wife and living in River Oaks.

In the past, I had suggested to Lottie Mae several times that we take Andy for a weekend, and she had declined. I inquired again that day. Lottie Mae called me into the kitchen to talk in private. She said, that on her death bed, Fritz's first wife had asked that she get a Bible, lay her hand on it and swear that she would never leave Andy alone in the same room with Fritz. Lottie Mae said that she complied with her wishes and that she would never break her promise.

I asked her why she didn't want Fritz in the same room with Andy. She told me she couldn't talk about that. It seemed my heart began to flutter a bit and my knees felt a tad weak. I thought, "My God, what is this all about." I was very quiet all the way home, as I imagined a million awful reasons why his first wife didn't want Fritz left alone with Andy.

The Burning Stump

Sometimes when Fritz wanted to be alone, he would go to his property down the street where he had an elaborate shop. The morning after the visit with his retarded son, Fritz went down the street to his hideaway. About two hours after he left, I looked in that direction, and saw smoke rising above the trees. I didn't think too much about it, since I figured Fritz could take care of any problems there.

In about thirty minutes, I heard a fire truck and from the window I could see it parked in front of his house. In about fifteen minutes, Fritz came stomping into the house. He was furious with the fire department. He had been trying to burn out an enormous stump of a diseased tree he had cut down. They put out the fire and threatened to arrest him. That wasn't the end of the burning stump. It certainly was the bane of my existence for the entire summer. It was as if Fritz had never heard the fire department's warnings to him. He became obsessed with the stump. Early the next morning, he was right down there burning the stump. I hurried down the street to try to persuade him to put out the fire. Simply put, he just ignored me, except for, "Woman, go home." In about an hour, I saw the red fire engine peeking through the trees, and again, Fritz came stomping home.

Over the summer, every few days he returned to the stump. He went to bed talking about the stump, and it was the first thing he thought about in the morning. His face carried a look of determination during those weeks. The fire department appeared another three or four times and threatened to send the police. Every time they came, they stayed about fifteen minutes. Fritz said they were just visiting, and they had become friends. I could see that Fritz's patience was wearing thin. Then, along about October, the stump was finally burned out and he sought out another project.

TAIL FEATHERS

In the spring of 1982 several families of pigeons came to roost on the capitals at the top of our front columns. In no time at all we had a nasty mess on our porch and columns. Fritz was very upset with the pidgeons. He hollered and threw things at them, but they just wouldn't go away. I guess it was the final straw, when one morning he brought in the newspaper that was spattered with pigeon doo. He said he'd had enough of that mess out front, and he had an idea for chasing off the pigeons.

He was out the door, and when he returned he sported a new Daisy air rifle. He stationed himself in the antique blue rocker and waited for the pigeons. I was appalled. A heated argument ensued, where he tried to convince me that he wouldn't hurt the birds. He said he would only hit their tail feathers. Well, there was no removing him from the front porch. I was very irritated with him. He spent several hours a day in the rocking chair with his B B gun. His concentration was equal to, or greater than, that which he gave to the burning stump.

The neighborhood policemen stopped to inquire why Fritz was spending so much time on the front porch in the rocker, and what about the gun? In the past he had brought them in for coffee. He did invite them in, and it was then I realized that they had thought the gun was real. Certainly, he was the picture of a rugged individualist, sitting in his rocker, holding the rifle upright with the butt resting on the porch. After four or five weeks, I realized that the pigeons were gone. I never saw a dead or wounded bird, but I did see a few tail feathers.

We only had about five large parties at our place. The one I remember most vividly was a birthday party I gave for Fritz. I hired a Dixieland jazz band. It was a warm June night, and the music could be heard all over the neighborhood. I guess there must have been about seventy-five people there. It was a loud and spirited party.

Midway through the party, Fritz and I were visiting with about a dozen friends in the breakfast room and kitchen when a large rat appeared on the counter. It all happened so fast that I really can't tell you how long Fritz and the rat went at it. The counter is long and curved. I just saw Fritz with his enormous hands swatting at the rat. The guests got very quiet, except for a few gasps. Fritz kept bashing the rat, and things on the counter went flying. Then the rat was at a dead end, at the end of the counter. There were about a dozen glasses of Baccarat crystal there. Fritz had it out with the rat right there, and all of the crystal was smashed to smithereens. Fritz held up the rat, and pinched off its head. I couldn't stand it. I just left the room.

Rachel Anne

It was a hot August afternoon, in the nineties, with ninety percent humidity. Fritz and I were on the front courtyard painting iron lawn furniture, when there came a chirpy little, "Hello." A pretty face was peeking through the iron gate. Her eyes were large, and pale blue, and tired-looking, and she looked to be in her fifties. Her skin was sun-wrinkled, and her hair was bleached yellow-blonde, and rolled up in pink plastic curlers. Her lips were tight, and painted fire engine red. Her cheeks were smudged with red rouge spots. I guess one would say that she had seen her day. She was definitely down on her luck, but she looked as if she were still holding onto a little bit of living. Even so, there was a certain sweetness that flowed from her.

She wore a pink silk georgette dress under a raggedy, knee-length, raccoon coat and high heels. I thought she looked a little bit like a peach faced love bird.

"Isn't that coat kind of warm on a hot day like this ?" I asked.

"No, but I sure could use a cold drink," she said.

I was drinking iced tea, and Fritz, a beer. "Would you care for an iced tea or a coke?" I asked.

Very matter-of-factly, she said, "No, but I'll take one of those Lone Stars."

Fritz said, "Sweetheart, go get . . . what's your name, Honey ?"

She said, "Rachel Anne."

Fritz said, "Liz, go get Rachel Anne a Lone Star."

I returned with the beer for Rachel Anne and we invited her into the house to cool off. She declined the invitation, preferring to sit on the porch and drink her beer. That took less than five minutes.

She carried a large old tattered leather purse. The zipper was broken and it overflowed with dirty, wrinkled papers. Later on Fritz said, "That purse she was carrying looked like a country landlord's purse."

After she finished her beer Fritz said, "Rachel Anne, honey, where are you going?" She said she was going to the store to buy some groceries. Fritz offered to take her, and she quickly accepted his offer with some excitement in her voice.

They were gone a good two hours. She had directed him to Safeway on West Gray. He waited in the truck for about forty-five minutes while she shopped. Then he went to investigate. She was taking her sweet time, and really didn't want any help with her shopping. Later, we figured she was just cooling off under the weight of that raccoon coat.

As long as it took, she came away with only one large bag of groceries. She bought only canned goods, no perishables.

Rachel Anne refused a ride to her place. When they returned home, she looked so pleased when Fritz helped her down out of the truck and said, "Be careful, Honey." She smiled just a little smile.

Abruptly she put down her sack and said, "Mr. Becker, I'll take another Lone Star." She drank her beer, took up her sack, and took off walking toward downtown. Fritz seemed pleased to have done the little favor for Rachel Anne, but said, "I never thought it was going to take all afternoon, and I couldn't get her to take off that Goddamned fur coat. It made me hot just looking at her."

We didn't see Rachel Anne for about a month. Then one day she appeared at the gate in her pink dress and raccoon coat and rang the bell. We went to the door, and very distinctly she said, "I want to go to the store, and to Walgreen's." She wouldn't come in, but waited at the gate.

It was another long shopping trek, and it took the better part of the afternoon. Again, she bought only canned goods. She refused Fritz's offer of a ride to her place. We wondered where she lived. She was very secretive, so we honored her privacy and didn't pry.

After about six or eight months, it occurred to us that Rachel Anne always visited us right after the first of each month. It occurred to me that perhaps her visits might coincide with Social Security checks that she might be receiving.

When we planned to be out of town we told Rachel Anne, so as not to disrupt her schedule and disappoint her. Sure enough, the next month she would be there ringing our doorbell, right after the first of the month.

As a matter of fact, Fritz had come to look forward to her visits. When we hadn't seen her for awhile, he'd say, "I wonder where Rachel Anne is, she hasn't been by for awhile. Do you suppose she might be sick?" We, very affectionately, referred to her as, "the peach-faced love bird."

One day we were on the courtyard planting flowers when Rachel Anne came by, wearing her raccoon coat. She was enamored with the flowers, pink periwinkles, and she ooooed and aaaahed over them. She wanted to know all about them, including their care. She said, "You know, I love flowers, but I never did have any. Pink is my favorite color. Would you give me one of those?"

Of course we would, and when they returned from grocery shopping, and after she drank her Lone Star, Fritz packed up a half-dozen plants, and she was on her way.

The regular shopping trips occurred right after the first of the month, and continued for about three years. Funny, even though we had known Rachel Anne for that long, we felt as if we really didn't know her any better now than on our first visit. That must have been the way she wanted it.

One evening on the local news, it was reported that an unidentified woman had been fatally shot in the area of White Oak Bayou, near downtown. The shooting had occurred in a place where a number of homeless people camped out. We were startled and speechless. The description given sounded identical to Rachel Anne, right down to the pink dress and raccoon coat.

The next day on the morning news it was reported that the police had arrested and taken into custody a man who had allegedly murdered a woman on the previous day at White Oak Bayou. He had attempted to cash a Social Security check made out to Rachel Anne Ryder.

We hurried down to the bayou, which was a mile or so away. There was an assortment of very large cardboard boxes that were covered with graffiti. There were clotheslines strung about, with clothes hung out to dry. There was a barbecue pit. Yes, people definitely lived here, whether we chose to believe it or not. We did not know that there were this many people down on their luck.

We were looking for someone who could tell us something about Rachel Anne. We passed the first box, and were on our way to the second box, when we were struck with the reality of the situation.

Fritz and I looked at each other, with tears brimming up in our eyes. There, outside the box was a beautiful little garden of pink periwinkles. Unmistakably, this was the place that Rachel Anne had called home.

In a few days there appeared on the news a report of a positive identification of Rachel Anne's murderer. Forensic evidence had shown that a hair taken from the suspect's clothing indeed matched one that was plucked from Rachel Anne's raccoon coat.

It was all too sad. On the way home we just talked about Rachel Anne. We wondered if she might have always worn the raccoon coat because she was protecting it from thieves, and was afraid to leave it in her box.

Yes, we were going to miss the "peach-faced love bird."

A Plan To Kill

In mid October there was a trip to the beach house that stands out very vividly in my mind. It was quite a lovely weekend, and just before leaving, we took a long walk on the beach, hand in hand, and once again Fritz proclaimed his love for me. It was dusk when we left for Houston. On the drive back, I admired the moonlight as it shone on the fall crops in the fields.

After a long silence, Fritz said, "Have you ever considered killing anyone?"

The question really jolted me. I said, "No, of course not."

He went on to say, "You know, I very carefully planned to kill Andy (his retarded and blind son). I had everything assembled that I needed to accomplish it. My planning was so deliberate and meticulous that there was no *way* I would have been caught. I still don't know why I didn't carry it out . . . and I'm sorry that I didn't."

He stared straight ahead with his jaw set and avoided looking at me for the rest of the trip home. My heart beat fast. I was stunned, and the questions that I wanted to ask just stuck in my throat. I never mentioned the conversation again. Later, I connected the talk Lottie Mae had with me (regarding the promise she had made to Fritz's first wife), to Fritz's confession on the ride home from the beach house.

A SUMMER HOLIDAY ABROAD

In spring of 1983 we departed on a five-month trip to Europe.

That first morning in London we met an English couple in the hotel lobby, and accepted an invitation to breakfast with them. The four of us spent the day sightseeing and cruising on the Thames.

Except for our reservations on the Orient Express, we did not make any hotel or travel reservations. We spent about a month and a half traveling around England and Ireland. We had purchased Eurail passes, and just jumped off the train when we came to a place that looked interesting. We visited Oxford, Stratford-on-Avon, Lemington Spa, Dublin, Edinburgh and many small towns in England, Scotland and Ireland.

The most romantic and delightful town in our travels was Bath, in England. It is nestled down in a deep valley, with the river Avon running through it. The town abounds with eighteenth century architecture, and there are brightly-colored flowers everywhere. We spent more than two weeks there, during which time it was sunny and brisk. We found a friendly little sidewalk cafe in the square, next to the abbey.

Almost every afternoon we talked, laughed, and sipped tea with the locals there. We received a number of invitations to dinner, and accepted a few of them. One lady entertained us in her early sixteenth century home named "Two Penny Cottage." We visited the museums, walked along the river Avon, and toured the Roman baths.

Also, we spent a long afternoon with a couple who resided at The Royal Crescent. This was a treat. It is said to be the most celebrated example of eighteenth century Georgian architecture in the world. High tea was served, with many different foods, and the best scones I've ever eaten.

Such a beautiful town, with such beautiful people, and so we departed from Bath with some regrets. We could imagine ourselves living there, and we talked quite a lot about that. Fritz said, "I think this would be a great place to live. I could distance myself from that miserable family of mine." We looked at a flat at The Royal Crescent that was for sale, and gave it very serious consideration.

On the train, we followed the coastline to Edinburgh. We found a quaint old hotel where we settled in. During the days we traipsed around the town and we would come to rest at the hotel's friendly pub in the late afternoons. There were always interesting people to talk to, and sometimes we carried our afternoons well into the evening, including dinner. We were there four or five days and on the last day we walked up the very steep Royal Mile, with its collection of wonderful shops. We bought some hand-knitted sweaters for my daughters, a herringbone tweed coat and a plaid wool hat for Fritz.

We took the train back to London, and stayed there for a week. We spent half of the days sightseeing and the rest of the time we spent at The Victoria and Albert Museum. We took a day to just loll around the hotel before we began one of the most luxurious parts of our journey.

We boarded the Orient Express at Victoria Station in London, and made our way to the dining car. The train had been restored to its original luxurious interior from the nineteen-twenties. Everything was sparkling. There was polished brass everywhere, Lalique lamps, and tables spread with white linen tablecloths and Lalique vases with fresh flowers.

We struck up an acquaintance with the couple across the aisle. He owned an art gallery in London. He and his fiancee were on their way to Paris for the weekend. They joined us for Bloody Marys before lunch. There was a noteworthy French chef on board. We lingered over a delicious lunch for several hours. The remainder of the afternoon we spent listening to the rhythm of the rails, while we watched the French countryside pass by.

Everyone dressed for dinner, and many appeared in nineteen-twenties attire. It was very festive, as we drank, talked and mingled with the other passengers up and down the length of the car.

We made the very elaborate dinner last almost as long as lunch. Then we sipped brandy and visited with our friends for an hour or so. Around eight o'clock it turned into a jazzy affair. Dixieland jazz and live piano music could be heard coming from the end of the car. Sure enough, there was a piano, and the drinks flowed, while the party got louder. We retired to our sleeping compartment around eleven o'clock. I was enchanted with the novelty of sleeping on the train. It was rather cozy, and in a few minutes I was lulled to sleep by the motion of the train.

I awakened in the morning, pulled back the curtain, and what, to my wondering eyes should appear, but a glorious sun rising over the majestic snow-capped Alps. I was mesmerized, motionless, and my breath was momentarily taken away. I don't believe I've ever awakened to such a splendid sight. After a few minutes I awakened Fritz to show him the dramatic view of the mountains that surrounded us. I started to say something and he interrupted with, "Hush, Hush," as he gently put his finger to my lips. Such a sensuous moment, and together, in silence we watched the sun rise over the mountain peaks.

We spent a week in Vienna. We sat outside at the coffee houses on the cobblestone square and drank quite a lot of coffee, and visited with people from around the world. We spent a lot of time at the museums, and also went to see the Lippizan stallions perform.

We were on our way to Venice from Vienna, on the train, and gazing at the scenery, when Fritz said, "What do you call those black things out there in the fields ?" I was alarmed. I was disturbed, and scared. I only said, "Cows, you mean the cows?"

And Fritz said, "Yes."

My mind went crazy. I thought, "Was it a small stroke, a brain tumor, a neurological disease, like Alzheimer's?" I connected the two occasions that Fritz forgot to meet me in the lobby of our London hotel. That was uncharacteristic of him. I felt helpless, and could see my world falling apart. I decided I would take him to a neurologist as soon as we returned home. For the remainder of our trip, I offered up many intense silent prayers.

We stayed for a week in Venice, where we rode along the canals in the gondolas, ate some great Italian food, and enjoyed the impressive ancient architecture.

After Venice, we spent several weeks in Florence viewing the incredible art. It was just impossible to see everything that should be seen, in just two weeks. We decided that we would have to return when we could stay for a month.

Rome was a delight, with its high spirit. It was loud and busy, with many motorcycles and motor scooters. It was easy to get caught up in its liveliness. We walked a lot, and spent a whole afternoon tramping around the ruins of the Coliseum. Fritz was in complete awe of the structure. One day we spent shopping, and had several custom suits tailored for Fritz. I bought a beautiful manicure set in a leather case.

We flew from Rome to Athens where we stayed for a few days. We visited the Parthenon, the most exciting part of our visit. It was named "Temple of Athena Polias," and was built in 447-438 B.C. and represents the culmination of the Doric, Classical style of architecture. There was so much history surrounding that spot that we spent most of the two days there.

We took a cab from Athens to the Port of Piraeus, where we boarded the cruise ship Stella Oceanis. We sailed south and east to the Cyclades in the Aegean, a group of about thirty islands. We visited about a dozen islands, each of which had its own flavor, and certainly I could not pick a favorite. The whole month that we spent in the Greek islands was a delight. We had expected that it would be very pleasant, but it was more, much more. It was the most exotic part of our trip.

The cruise ship did not go to some of the islands we wished to visit, so we took the ferry to those. We spent a week on Mykonos. Upon approaching the island one sees hills of dazzling white cubic houses with bright blue and green shutters and doors. All of the buildings are whitewashed twice a year. There are about 300 tiny churches. We spent a lot of time walking around the island. There were little gardens of hibiscus, pink oleanders, acacia, eucalyptus and pepper trees. There were windmills scattered on the hillsides. The atmosphere is very cosmopolitan, with hotels, taverns and discotheques. We spent some time down close to the dock at a sidewalk cafe, drinking beer and visiting with tourists.

After leaving Mykonos, we visited Delos, which is a mile-and-a-half west of Mykonos. We spent a memorable evening watching the sun set from the top of Mt. Kynthos, which is 368 feet high. In terms of historical significance, the island abounds in riches. We visited the Hieron of Apollo, the

Statue of Apollo, the "Great" Temple of Apollo, Temple of the Athenians, the Sanctuary of Artemis, the Monument of the Bulls and many other historic sites.

We visited Syros, Tinos and Andros. On Andros there were beautiful green hills and many vineyards laden with fruit. We went on to Samos. It was a different kind of beauty; mountainous and wooded with an abundance of superb scenery. We visited Paros, where we saw what is said to be the most beautiful church in the Aegean. It is the Panagia Ekatontapyliani, or Our Lady of the Hundred Gates. We also visited the marble quarries.

Other islands we visited were Rhodes, Kos and Thira. The month we spent in the islands just flew by. They were glorious, and the waters of the Aegean are a deep blue-green. Now, when I wish to conjure up a scene of serene beauty in my mind's eye, I always think of those incredible Greek islands and the surrounding Aegean sea.

We left the serene and peaceful green waters of the Aegean and the azure blue skies with some regrets, but with promises to return. We flew from Athens to Paris, where we would spend a week or so before returning home.

Paris was a delight. We walked a lot, talked a lot, and spent a great deal of time sitting outside at the sidewalk cafes. Most especially, we enjoyed The Rodin Museum and The Jeu de Pomme, both very small museums with impressive collections. Also, The Louvre took the greater part of three days, and certainly was well worth the little bit of time afforded it. Indeed, it would have been easy to have devoted a whole summer to seeing the Louvre. We spent some time walking on the Left Bank, and an afternoon at Notre Dame Cathedral. Paris was beautiful. Paris was fun. And Paris *is for lovers!*

Several hours into the flight from Paris to Houston, Fritz said, "Please give me one of those." He was referring to a piece of fruit in my tote bag, where there were two bananas and an orange. “One of the yellow ones, what do you call it ?”

All of the anxieties associated with the previous cow incident on the train returned. I thought, “What is wrong? What is wrong?” I was clearly frightened. All the way home I thought, “What doctors should we see? What is the disease? What is the prognosis? How can I live without him?” These relentless thoughts taunted me for the rest of the flight.

"There Is No Cure. There Is No Cure."

We arrived in Houston at the end of August, and as we stepped off the plane, an unwelcome wave of heat and humidity was in our faces. We learned that we had just missed Hurricane Alicia, which had hit Houston on August 18th.

It was pure joy being in our home again. Our garden was in full bloom with twenty-one crape myrtle trees, several dozen rose bushes, and lots of blue plumbago. Always, our garden was a source of peace for us, even if we had to view it from our breakfast room, due to the hot August Texas sun.

Our dogs were ecstatic to have us back. By now, we had two big Airedales and a black Labrador. I wondered if they thought we had abandoned them.

However, as good as it was to be home, a black cloud hung over me. Even our garden afforded me no peace. I found a referral for Fritz to a well-recommended geriatric psychiatrist in the medical center. The earliest appointment was a week away. During that time, it seemed I died a thousand little deaths as I tossed and turned the nights away.

There were no simple answers at the doctor, only a lot of history-taking and an appointment set for the next day with a neurologist. Over a period of three days, there was a battery of exhausting tests. Following, was another week of waiting, with the accompanying high anxiety, before we returned to the psychiatrist for the test results.

During that week, Fritz found a job to do. The hurricane had uprooted enormous live oak trees in River Oaks. There were large piles of fireplace-sized wood on the curbs. We spent the entire week hauling the wood in our pickup. The wood lasted us for more than five years. Fritz wanted it all. Thank heavens, it started to rain, for that ended the wood hauling.

Before the appointment for the test results, I telephoned the doctor. Fritz had always driven fast, but now he drove faster-than-fast and sometimes didn't stop at stop signs or red lights. I asked the doctor to recommend to Fritz that he discontinue driving.

The doctor called both of us into his office. He proceeded to say that although there was no conclusive test for Alzheimer's Disease, from all of the available tests, it appeared that this was the diagnosis. Then he said, "There is no cure." And it echoed loudly in my ears, "There is no cure, no cure, no cure. *Oh, God*!" He went on to say that it was a progressive, degenerative disease, ending in death. There is a gradual loss of all intellectual functions. This is known as dementia. He said thinking, remembering and reasoning are severely affected, and eventually the patient is unable to function, becomes incontinent, and unable to talk. Then the doctor spoke with each of us privately.

Without a word, sadly, we walked hand in hand to our car. With a mean look on his face, Fritz took the car keys, and very reluctantly and deliberately, placed them in my hand.

I drove, and we rode home in silence. I always knew when Fritz did not wish to have a conversation, and this was definitely one of those times.

At home, Fritz went directly to the telephone. He called The Houston Club and made reservations for dinner in one hour. Very quietly, he came from behind me and carefully turned me around and said, "Sweetheart, we're going to The Houston Club for dinner in one hour." Then there was a long and tender kiss, and he said, "You do what you need to do. I'm going to play the piano for awhile."

At The Houston Club we ordered drinks before dinner. Since the visit with the doctor, there had been no discussion of Fritz's devastating diagnosis. He reached across the table, took both of my hands, and held them firmly in his own. He said, "Darling, you know that I love you deeply, and there is absolutely nothing that I would change about our lives. Now, you heard what the doctor said. Apparently I have the same debilitating disease that affected my mother. This development is very disturbing to me. Now, Sweetheart, I want our lives to continue just as if we hadn't even heard the doctor today. I'd like for you to put all of that out of your mind. I want our focus to be on living. I realize that this is an unusual request, but it is my way of coping, and the only way I know.

Also, when I get like my mother was, I want you to take those necessary steps to see to it that I don't hang around some nursing home for years. That's not where I want to be. Now, one of the reasons I married you was that you're such a gutsy woman. I sincerely hope that you will have the courage to carry out my wishes. I do not intend to discuss this with my family, and I don't want you to. If you want to tell your family, that's all right with me. As you know, I don't consider my family part of my life anyway. I haven't for a long time . . . since way before we met."

By this time, the tears took over, and streamed uncontrollably down my cheeks. Fritz said, "Sweetheart, put your chin up, and let's pretend. I don't ever want to speak of this again. The last thing I want to say is that I am so very sorry that you have to carry this burden.

I love you in a way that I've never loved a woman. I don't believe I really knew how to love a woman until I met you, and you made it so easy. Now, Darling, let's dance."

TEARS ON THE AUBUSSON

Every morning I awakened to the sweet smell of freshly-brewed coffee that drifted up and into our bedroom. This was the best part of the day, and I would lay very still and inhale the sweet aroma. Today, I yawned, opened my eyes, and looked through the intricate patterns of the antique lace curtains that we had bought in Dublin. The sun was just coming up, and I could see the dramatic Houston skyline, which was about a mile away.

Soon, I smelled the bacon. Since we had first met, almost every morning, Fritz had brought me breakfast in bed. He loved doing this, and I was more than a willing and happy recipient of his offerings.

Quietly, I watched the leaves flutter from the stately sycamore tree outside our bedroom window. An ominous feeling crept into my consciousness, and it was then I realized that although the sun was shining, it was far from being a sunny day. Yesterday's seemingly callous words of the doctor came to me. "It is a progressive, degenerative disease, ending in death. There is no cure." I thought, "Death, I'm not even sure right now that I know what that means." Certainly, I didn't know the manifestations of a progressive, degenerative disease, and was not at all prepared for the drastic and hideous changes that were about to take place in our lives. Large tears erupted from my eyes and flowed down my cheeks, as I groaned and turned my face into my pillow.

I heard the jingle of our dog's tags as she ran up the stairs to announce breakfast. Quickly, I composed myself, wiped the tears from my face and tried to bury my depressing thoughts.

Fritz was smiling and happy and said, "Good morning, beautiful. Are you hungry?" And it was just like any other day. I lied, and said I was hungry, and ate all of the breakfast that he had so lovingly prepared.

We spent all of the morning planting thirty burgundy-colored mums. Fritz attacked the project with his usual enthusiasm. When we finished our gardening, we sat on the terrace and admired the fruits of our labor. The black dog lay beside us, soaking up the sunshine. The burgundy mums looked terrific with the cascading bushes of blue plumbago. Again, I returned to reality, and was reminded that this was *not* forever. How could that be? Just yesterday, I had thought it was. In one day, my world began to crack and fall apart. There was no joy in our garden and it was different than before, the difference being, I did not see the future there.

Fritz suggested that we scrub up and go for a picnic lunch in the park. Iris, the black Labrador, liked to run in the woods, so we took her along. We picked up barbecue sandwiches at Otto's Barbecue on Memorial Drive and drove down the road a couple of miles to the Houston Arboretum in Memorial Park.

We drove about a block into the woods and parked our car. We walked deeper into the woods to the spot we had come to call our own. This part of the woods was very private, and seemed miles from civilization. It was untended and on the wild side. The trees were thick and very tall. We spread our blanket on a bed of leaves and lay down. We lay in each others arms, and Fritz held me very close for a long time. We did not speak. Perhaps we were both wondering how much time there was left for us. I was. For that time, the world simply did not exist. We fell fast asleep, watching the clouds float by the treetops, and listening to the songs of the birds.

When we awakened, the bag with our sandwiches was gone. We asked Iris about it. She ran away with her head down and her tail between her legs.

Every November Fritz spent hours cleaning and polishing his hunting rifles. He packed his survival kit and took off with his hunting buddies for our hunting lodge in Salida, Colorado, for a couple of weeks. Now, I wondered if it was safe for him to still do that.

Right then and there, I formed a policy which would be important in guiding me in directing his life in the days ahead. I would allow him to be his own fiercely independent self, as long as it did not become highly dangerous. Why shouldn't he do all the things he was accustomed to doing? And hadn't he made it perfectly plain to me that he wished his life to continue just as it had been before?

So be it. I would not stand in the way. Hadn't he always lived his life just a little close to the edge? Who was I to change his modus operandi? Actually, I don't believe he would have allowed my interference, anyway. So, it seemed to me that I had just made an important decision.

The morning Fritz was leaving for his annual hunting trip to Colorado, I helped him pack his bags, and he threw in the wool stocking cap I had knitted for him. That pleased me.

His hunting buddy was to arrive in forty-five minutes. Since everything was in order, I disappeared into the bathroom to have a bath. In about ten minutes the doorbell rang. Shortly thereafter I stepped out of the tub. In fact, I stepped out of the tub at the precise moment that a huge hunter in an orange cap burst into my bathroom. I didn't even have the security of a towel. My God, such an embarrassing moment. The hunter disappeared quickly.

In about ten minutes, Fritz appeared. He tried to persuade me to come out to see them off. I was sitting on the potty, still naked, and crying. Fritz didn't know what had happened. He said that Jim really wanted to see me. I told him that Jim had seen all of me, and all he was going to see that day. He begged me to dress and come out, but I absolutely refused. Right then and there, I didn't want to ever see him again. That is how we said our good-byes, in the bathroom, Fritz in his red-and-black buffalo-checked shirt, and me, without even a towel.

As soon as they were out the door, I dashed down the stairs to be sure that Fritz had locked the door. Then I went into the living room, flopped on the aubusson couch, and burst into tears. The tears had nothing to do with the hunter in my bathroom. It had been several months since my world had begun to quake, and there had been no time for tears. How could I cry, when Fritz had pleaded with me to participate in his denial? On the face of things, I would say he was doing a masterful job of controlling his emotions. Now, the events of the last two months were upsetting my equanimity and ripping out my insides, from top to bottom, as the tears flowed onto the aubusson.

I was still without my clothes, which didn't seem at all important right now, except that I was beginning to shiver. I used the many needlepoint pillows to warm my body, stuffing them in here and there. The black dog nestled her face close by my head. The Texaco Saturday afternoon opera came on, "La Traviata," by Verdi. Iris stayed with me, her head next to mine. I don't know why, but after awhile, the black dog began to cry.

I lay on the couch for the entire afternoon, with Iris on the floor beside me. I tossed and turned. I moaned and groaned and boo-hooed, and wondered if I would ever have the mind to rise up again. My eyes were swollen and my nose was sore. In short, I was a mess, and I remember thinking that I had never been so full of pain.

From the couch I watched the light of day fade into the peripheral pink tinges of the sunset. Darkness came quickly, as I watched a blurred misty moon rise high in the sky.

Although I hadn't eaten since breakfast, I was not hungry. In fact, my appetite had been on the wane for the last couple of months. I conjured up a vision of the contents of the refrigerator. There was nothing there that was worth a trip to the kitchen. Besides that, I was weak and exhausted and wasn't even sure I could make it to the kitchen. When I had just made the decision to sleep on the couch, Iris began asking to go outside. I simply had to drag myself off the couch to walk the black dog. Certainly, I didn't want her urinating on the antique Serapi rug, but on second thought, right now, what the hell difference did it make anyway?

I threw on some clothes and took my remote security alarm from the top drawer of the Chippendale chest in the foyer, and Iris and I were out the door. Iris relieved herself and then took off down the sidewalk with a big smile on her face. After cruising the neighborhood, we returned home. I believe we both felt a little better, and I was glad that I had a dog.

When we returned, I put on a record, an opera by Puccini, "Suor Angelica." I turned the volume up high, so that the music took control of my unconscious self, and the pain seemed to melt away.

The black dog and I climbed the grand, winding staircase, and paused on the landing to admire the crystal chandelier. I looked down into the large foyer at our art gallery, and reminisced back to the days when we had hung it. Actually, it had been four days of pure hell. Our ceilings are very high, so

Fritz spent a lot of time on the ladder. I directed the operation. Perhaps that was the problem. Sometimes, we called in Pat, to help lift a painting. There was almost continuous hollering, bickering and fighting. Pat hated it and would say, "God, I'll be glad when this gallery is up there, Mrs. Becker. I don't think I can stand much more of this. I don't understand it. When I hang my pictures, I just puts a nail in the wall, hits it, and says, 'God bless.'"

There was a collision of our respective perfectionisms. Fritz became exasperated with me and said, "What do you mean move it three millimeters to the left? What the hell difference does three millimeters make? I didn't know that I was married to a crazy prima donna. When you asked me to help you hang some pictures, I thought that meant a couple of hours work. I've been on this goddamned ladder for four days."

We had just three more pictures to hang, when Fritz jumped off the ladder, right onto our tomcat's tail. The cat went berserk. He tore into Fritz's legs, digging his claws in deep. Fritz retaliated by kicking the hell out of the cat. The cat landed on a Queen Anne desk, and crashed an eighteenth century Delft vase into hundreds of pieces. Over Fritz's loud protestations, I took him to the emergency room, where twenty-seven stitches were put in his legs.

I stood on the landing, and thought of that four-day fiasco, as I looked down into the foyer with all the works of art. That was our first and last fight, and it was a big one. I smiled.

I felt weak, fragile and emotionally spent. I climbed into bed, lay down, and closed my eyes. I thought of the box of truffles under the bed. I crawled under, pulled it out, got back into bed, and switched on "Saturday Night Live."

The truffles were a nightly ritual, and Fritz was keeper of the candy. He would take a truffle from the box and meticulously feed it to me. It was a silent ceremony that lasted around ten minutes. If I started to talk, he would frown. If the phone rang, it went unanswered.

I snuggled into the pillows, pulled up the covers, and sunk my teeth into the rich, smooth chocolate. It was divine. My thoughts returned to the grim outlook for Fritz's health. The tears began to flow again, and I didn't see or hear the television. I only know that as the tears flowed, and in robotic fashion, four truffles disappeared.

The following two weeks were difficult for me. I did not answer the telephone, and only once did I leave the house, and that was to visit The Alzheimer's Association's office. I picked up a pile of literature there, and devoured it immediately. Then, I burned all of it in the fireplace. I was now more depressed than ever, and again, the tears flowed. And again, the black dog cried.

Seeking some solace, one afternoon I bundled up and sat in our garden, with a cup of hot tea. I couldn't seem to find the peace and beauty that had only recently existed here. Every direction my mind took, frustration confronted me. I prayed and prayed. I cried and cried, and once, I even screamed. Thank God, no one responded to my scream, only the black dog. She barked.

Always, I had felt somewhat in control of my destiny, but here was something I could not begin to cope with. All avenues seemed to lead to a dead end. I didn't remember ever having been in a position where there seemed to be no possible chance of a resolution.

To accompany my perfectly miserable self, the November rains came. The two weeks were interminable. I felt as if I had been overwhelmed by a tidal wave. As I floated, I felt as if I were being propelled along inside that wave.

It was a Sunday evening when Fritz returned from the Colorado mountains, and I had just given myself a good talking-to regarding the game of pretend that I was obliged to resume. It seemed as if he had been gone for a year. We were ecstatic. We sat in the living room in front of the fire, and sipped a little Remy Martin. Fritz proudly presented his gift to me. Always, it was the same, a handful of pretty little rocks. I was touched. Today, there's a little silver box on the piano, filled with rocks from the mountain. There's also three little rocks Fritz picked up at the Coliseum in Rome. Occasionally, I sit on the aubusson with the silver box, touching and caressing each one, and reminiscing about the feelings that accompanied these gifts. I feel closer to his soul. They were given with love. And they were given with passion.

Just before we retired, Fritz handed me the front page of a Colorado newspaper. The headlines read, "HUNTER LOST ON MOUNTAIN." It went on to say, "Fritz Becker, of Houston, Texas was lost on the mountain, near Salida, for more than a day. A posse of twenty-five men searched all day for Mr. Becker." It was a two column article. Fritz said he hadn't been worried at all and didn't know what all the hullabaloo was about. He said he had strayed off the path, but he knew that he could find his way back if he climbed to the top of the mountain and looked down.

He did that, and then walked right down to the cabin. They said in the article that over the years many men had been lost on that mountain this time of the year, and had frozen to death. God, I was speechless. Then I had a most ghastly thought, "Wouldn't it be less painful to freeze to death on the mountaintop, than slowly lose one's mind and all one's bodily functions?" Without a doubt, I knew the answer to that question.

The next day there came an urgent, loud knocking on our door. It was the tenant down the street. She was hollering,

"Mr. Becker, Mr. Becker, come help me! Mama's stuck in the bathtub!"

Being a friendly landlord, Fritz hurried down the street with her. He was gone about a half hour. When he returned, he could hardly stop laughing long enough to tell me what had happened. Yes, Mama was indeed stuck in the old-fashioned bathtub. Fritz said it hadn't been easy, and that for a while he thought he was going to have to call his friends at the fire department. After many attempts, finally, he had to get behind her, put his arms under her arms and around her chest and PULL. Fritz said, "There was a big sucking, slurping noise, like what a toilet plunger makes, (Fritz imitated the sound) and she came loose."

A Night at The Opera

Although he still enjoyed his Lone Star with meals, it seemed that Remy Martin appeared more and more frequently throughout the day. I could never tell when Fritz had had too much to drink. His days were filled with obsessive, very hard physical work, with only a few minutes' pause for meals.

That particular October evening was opening night at the opera, always a festive affair. The guard at The Federal Building always allowed us to park in Fritz's old C.I.A. space. That was nice, since it was just a few steps from Jones Hall.

There were limousines, lovely ladies in beautiful dresses, and dashing gentlemen. We arrived about fifteen minutes early so we could soak up the ambiance and exchange greetings with a few of our friends.

I wore a stunning long black silk dress, by Oscar de la Renta, with a narrow, hip-hugging skirt that was split (front and back) from here to kingdom come. It had great bouffant elbow-length sleeves. I wore my opera length pearls and a deco Cartier diamond bracelet that was an unbelievable inch wide. "Sweetheart, you look like a flower. Look around you, now tell me, aren't you the most gorgeous woman at the opera tonight? You just look fit to kill." And then in a low saucy whisper he began to sing, "Ain't she sweet? See her coming down the street." And the old black magic returned.

At the opera Fritz promptly fell asleep, and went limp. Then the snoring began. It was low and loud and lewd. Quickly I jabbed him with my elbow and restored his respirations to normal, but only after he had uttered a loud, ludicrous snort. Oh God, I took a deep breath, wiggled my toes and squirmed in my seat. Should we stay or should we go? I felt badly about imposing this less-than-musical sideshow on our fellow opera-goers, many of whom we had briefly come to know.

Over the course of the evening, I had to relive that same snoring scenario three more times. My most dreaded fears did not materialize. Our friends did not ask us to leave. I considered that very gracious indeed.

In the past, we never left our seats before the last applause ceased. Tonight we did. Toward the end of the opera, Fritz's head plopped over, almost parallel with his shoulder, and remained there. Then, unannounced, Sweet-Heart-Pie toppled into the center aisle.

Jesus, Joseph and Mary! Remy Martin had taken its toll. He just sat there looking very stupid. Then a barrage of questions followed, "Where the hell am I, Sweetheart? Where is Remy Martin? Why are you so dressed up? Are we having guests? And, who are all those people clapping for ?"

"For you, Honey-Bun, for you." It was the end of an aria. I seized the opportunity to extricate myself from the bad scene. Somehow I escaped with him. It wasn't easy. I kind of half-dragged him, with little mincing steps (due to my narrow skirt and high heels). All the while, he was muttering something about Remy Martin and his ukulele. We made it up the long aisle, from way down front, while the lights were still down low. Thank God for that.

The cool night air and the walk to the truck revived him. I was startled by the realization that Fritz had the truck keys in his pocket. Instantly, I tried to conjure up a thoughtful solution that would enable a smooth transition of the keys to me without provoking my testy companion.

Diplomacy failed and the situation rapidly deteriorated. He looked mean. Unlocking the door on the passenger side, and like a thunderbolt, he bellowed out an order, "Get in the truck, woman!"

Very firmly, I said, "No, I'm NOT going to ride with you. You've had too much to drink. Now, Pleeeeeeeese, just let me have the keys, so I can drive us home."

In a sing-songy kind of voice he replied, "Oh now, Miss Big wants to put herself in the driver's seat, does she? And, in the driver's seat of *my big yellow truck.* NO, you're NOT driving. Now, get your ass up in there, so we can get the hell out of here. It's near eleven o'clock."

I thought, "May the Lord be with me and my spirit . . . and what's next? Is this the end of hearts and flowers?"

Generations of German ancestry were beginning to reveal themselves. My thoughts were punctuated by an outburst of passion. In a frenzy, he scooped me up and tossed me onto the seat of the truck. I gasped. My reaction to outrageous situations has always been to scream bloody murder. I uttered an ear-piercing, blood-curdling cry. Fritz crashed the door closed and at breakneck speed whipped around the rear of the truck and bounced onto the seat behind the wheel.

Midway through the scream, a disruption occurred. It was like a quake in the night. It took the form of a quick, heavy hand. I gasped as he anchored his enormous thick thumb inside my ear, and clamped his palm over my mouth to cut off my cries. He, very effectively, silenced me.

In a low, well-modulated voice he said, "Now Sweetheart, you know I would never hurt you. Don't you know that I love you dearly? Now relax. I just want you to turn off that goddamned noise."

Since his hand was still firmly pressed to my mouth, it seemed that any attempt to initiate another scream would have been futile. I felt weak and weary, and then there came a tapping on Fritz's window. Quickly, he released me. I sat up, prim and proper. It was Mr. Stoltzberg, the guard at the Federal Building, who used to exchange German ancestry stories with Fritz. "Mrs. Becker, do you need help?"

Fritz quickly answered for me. "No, Liz and I were just sitting here talking about the opera, and I was fastening her pearls that came undone."

Warily, the guard glanced across at me, for confirmation of this not-too-believable explanation, and said, "Mrs. Becker, are you sure everything is all right?"

I smiled sweetly and in a nonchalant voice said, "Oh yes, we just came from the opera. We're fine, but thank you for inquiring."

I don't believe he bought Fritz's story, but he bade us good evening and disappeared into the Federal Building.

My watch read eleven-fifteen. In a moderate voice, and with a great deal of finesse, once again I inquired, "I wonder if you would reconsider, and let me drive home?"

Oh my God. Fritz became electrified, and large sparks flew. "Oh you do wonder, do you? Well, that's the trouble with you. You wonder too much. Now, close your eyes, zip up your mouth, lie back, and I'll have you home in two minutes flat."

That was what frightened me. In a flash, I leaped from the truck and took off like a bat out of hell. I tore around the corner and down Smith Street, away from town, in my tight skirt and high heels. I had gotten a head start, but the big yellow truck quickly overtook me.

Thank God, the traffic was light. Several cars passed and I turned my face away. I pretended I belonged on Smith

Street, downtown, alone at night. On my right, I was passing Tranquillity Park. That made me smile.

Then came that unmistakable sound of the Chevy engine approaching from the rear. There was a slight screech of the brakes, and there it was in all its glory, the big yellow truck with the small decal on the window that read, "DON'T FUCK WITH MY TRUCK," and the simple blue-and-white bumper sticker that read, "OPERA." It certainly had a personality all its own. It stood up proudly on four huge oversized tires, and just in case we should fall off the side of a Colorado mountain cliff, it was equipped with a roll bar. The last significant feature was a gun rack, cradling a twelve-gauge shotgun, that glistened when the sun shone on it.

I pretended not to recognize the driver. He had become a mean old German. With my head tilted back, I inhaled deeply, and forged ahead . . . Adelante!

Soon, there came a loud cry. "Hey, you stuck-up Yankee bitch, where do you think you're going?"

"I'm going home, stupid," I said.

"Yeah, and you're going home with me, you crazy woman. Now, get your Yankee ass over here, right now. I mean it," he said.

I did not answer him. I was furious, but continued on my way. I concentrated on saving my breath. I was getting very tired. He continued to heckle me in a loud voice. After a few blocks I paused to take off my heels.

By now he had adjusted his speed to about five miles per hour in order to stay even with me. He didn't adjust his volume. There was still a stream of blaring commands: "Yankee bitch... Yankee bitch, get over here, or I'm coming after you!"

"No you're not. Go away. I'm NOT riding with you!" I said.

"You just think you're not. Now get the hell over here!" he said.

"If you stop the truck and give me the keys, and let me drive, I'll come over there," I said.

He said, "Oh you will, will you? Well, you just listen to me. When I give YOU the keys to my big yellow truck, that'll be a cold day in hell. Now get over here before you get arrested!"

I said, "Arrested, for what ? I'm not breaking any law. I'm minding my own business. It's you. You're the one being illegal. You're driving too slow, and you're hassling me. And what's more, you're disturbing the peace. Now, be nice, and go away!"

It was ten blocks from Jones Hall to home, about a mile. Oh God, how far had I come ? Halfway? Maybe.

I passed "Luther's Barbecue," "Harry's Kenya," and was now passing The Hyatt Regency Hotel on my left, and Allen Center on my right.

I was beginning to wonder if I could make it all the way without a rest. My feet hurt, my legs ached, and my stomach was starting to cramp. Several blocks ahead I could see "SPEC'S" big neon sign. That had become Fritz's favorite sign. It is Houston's party center and liquor store. I was three blocks from home.

Simultaneously, Fritz passed me and there came the flashing lights of the familiar blue Houston Police car. It was Officer Russell and his buddy. Over the years they had spent quite a few hours at our place, with Fritz, drinking coffee and swapping stories.

"Mrs. Becker, wasn't that your husband that just passed by?" inquired Officer Russell. I told him that it was, and that we had had a little disagreement. He told me that I shouldn't be out here on the street alone. He suggested that I get in their car and they would drive me home. It was a relief. I quickly got in.

They drove me the few blocks home. The big yellow truck was parked in the driveway, and the bedroom light was turned on. The officers escorted me to the door and rang the doorbell. After a moment Fritz came to the door in his robe. With a big smile and in a friendly voice he said, "Good evening, officers. Would you like to come in?"

Officer Russell replied, "No sir, but thank you. We are just returning your wife home."

Very sweetly, Fritz said, "Well, thank you . . . Hello, Sweetheart. Where've you been?"

"Darling, to the opera, of course," I replied.

TEA ROSE

Several years before he left home, Fritz began drinking heavily. He drank anything that resembled alcohol. Out of desperation, I gave away the entire contents of our liquor cabinet. He made due with his Lone Star beer. Shortly after the liquor disappeared, one evening, from our bed, I saw Fritz in the bathroom drinking something. He was chug-a-lugging my large bottle of Tea Rose cologne. I called the doctor immediately. Then I gave him Syrup of Ipecac, to induce vomiting. He vomited profusely. That was the last time that he ever drank anything from a bottle off my dresser.

During 1984 Fritz had at least a half dozen grease fires, while cooking breakfast. When we had purchased our security system, we also installed a fire alarm. It summoned the fire department in the event of a fire. After several calls to our house, one day the fire chief said, "We figured Mr. Becker was cooking breakfast again." During this period, Fritz also burned a ton of papers in the fireplace. God only knows what he burned, but on several occasions the smoke alarm sounded. He had forgotten to open the damper and the smoke quickly poured out and filled the house. It was dark and thick all over. When the fire department responded, Fritz told them that he was cleaning out his files. It was about then, that I told Pat we were going to have to watch him more carefully.

RUFUS

Summer came, and Fritz spent quite a lot of time piddling in the yard. One day I looked out and he was gone. I was terrified. The black dog was gone too. I jumped in the car and went looking for him. After forty-five minutes I found him in the Fourth Ward, a small black community about a mile away. He was sitting on the porch of a shotgun shack with Iris, visiting with an old black man named Rufus. He looked as if he were really enjoying himself. They invited me to join them, and for about a half hour, the three of us had a conversation. I gave Rufus our telephone number, so he could call me if Fritz came to call again. That turned out to be an intelligent thing to do, because he visited Rufus many more times.

A Chi Chi,
Drunk on Chinaberries

Often, in summer, we left the breakfast room door open for a little fresh air. One morning, while we were having coffee on the rear terrace, I returned inside the house for more coffee. Lo and behold, there was a sparrow flitting around the kitchen and breakfast room. There had been birds in the house before, but not like this one. I had forgotten to close off the inside doors, so the bird was loose in the rest of the house. Then it flew upstairs. Judging from the way it was flying, the bird seemed to have gone crazy. It moved fast and frantically around the room, hitting the walls. After an hour or so, we were successful in shooing it out the upstairs balcony doors.

When all was said and done, Fritz said, "That was a chi chi, and it was drunk on chinaberries. When I was a kid in Dallas, we had a chinaberry tree in our yard and the chi chis were always getting drunk on those china berries." Of course, there was a chinaberry tree next door, and as for the chi chis, I never heard a sparrow called a chi chi.

MARY RAE

During 1985 Fritz's memory suffered severely. It became obvious to me that he was rapidly losing his vocabulary. He would grope for simple words to complete a sentence. Sometimes, his reasoning was all off. While out to lunch one day, there was a young girl sitting next to us with her parents. Fritz whispered to me, "Do you see that girl over there? That's Mary Rae! She was in my high school class. That's her. I know it is!"

I replied, "Well, how is it that you're about forty years older than she is?"

We both just laughed, and Fritz said, "Yes, come to think of it, I guess that's not possible."

I can't tell you how much that conversation disturbed me. It confirmed to me, the doctor's words, "degenerative disease and there is a gradual loss of all intellectual functions." And I thought that yes, this is the beginning of the end.

THAT DAMNED PAT

Intermittently, Fritz would gently nag me about letting Pat go. His argument was that we didn't need a maid, that we could do it ourselves, and do it better. Lastly, we could have our home all to ourselves, without having to give up our privacy.

Then, some unusual things started happening on days Pat had been here. I found dirty dishes in the oven and in the dishwasher. There was scouring powder sprinkled into the otherwise clean bathtubs. Of course, Fritz was right there to incriminate Pat.

I spoke to Pat, and of course she wasn't responsible. Very good-naturedly, she said, "Mr. Becker just wants you all to himself." The incidents continued, and became more serious. The clothes in my closet were messed up and little things turned up cracked and broken.

The worst damage was a huge crack in the wash basin of a large antique Waterford crystal piece that had a matching pitcher. It was carefully placed where I could easily survey the damage. It was unbelievable that Fritz could do such a thing, but it was nevertheless true. I was crushed. Neither Pat nor I had even been in the guest bedroom where the basin sat on a dresser.

Without any accusations, I showed Fritz the damaged crystal basin. Lately, he had become a little cantankerous, so I didn't think it a good idea to challenge him, or even imply that he might be responsible.

"That damned Pat. We've got to get rid of her," he said.

Of course Pat stayed, and in the years ahead I credited her with the preservation of my sanity.

WANDERLUST

Since Fritz had started wandering off, I kept the big iron gate locked all the time. However, Fritz got around that. He just climbed over the fence. I always made sure he had his wallet in his pocket along with his name and address. He liked being outside so much, that I just couldn't lock him inside the house. He ran off many times, which caused me a great deal of aggravation and distress. My most dreaded memories are those when he took the car keys and escaped in the car. I would be on the verge of panic. His driver's license had expired long ago. When he ran off in the car, I would immediately call the police. They would find him and lead him home. He became easily disoriented, and when he got more than a couple of blocks from home, he became lost.

I spent a lot of time chauffeuring Fritz about. He bowled in three leagues, and attended a Rotary Club luncheon once a week. One hot August afternoon, I went to pick him up at the bowling alley. He was gone. I was so very frightened. It was out of our neighborhood, and the temperature was 98 degrees outside. I drove around for over an hour looking for him. Then I returned home to call the police.

Fritz was sitting on the front porch, and didn't know how he had gotten there. I started to cry. Later, I found a name and telephone number in his pocket. I called the number and found that this man had stopped and picked Fritz up about two miles from the bowling alley. The man reported that he had seen Fritz just trudging along in the heat, and had decided that he didn't look as if he belonged there. He said he had gotten Fritz's address out of his wallet.

My life was becoming increasingly more complicated, as well as frustrating. Everywhere I turned there was a brick wall. Sometimes my equanimity evaporated. When Fritz was gone, I would pace around the house, wringing my hands and boo-hooing.

Sometimes I would call my children and tell them all of the awful things Fritz was doing, like breaking things. I received absolutely no sympathy from any of them. Not one of them would believe a bad thing about Fritz. They thought he was *it*.

They only said, "Mother, you know you've always had a rich imagination. Fritz wouldn't do a thing like that." I was exasperated.

There is a row of very hardy Indian Hawthorn bushes along the rear of our house. I had noticed that the one on the corner had started to wither, and looked as if it might die. Then one day, I looked out to see Fritz boldly urinating on the Indian Hawthorn. He didn't understand at all why I was so furious. He paid no attention whatsoever, and continued his watering. Eventually the bush died.

Fritz's Bonus

One day we lunched at a popular restaurant on Montrose Boulevard. We went there often. As we were leaving, the owner followed us out onto the sidewalk. Then he tapped Fritz on the shoulder, and graciously said, "Excuse me sir, I wonder if you would mind returning our ashtrays and flatware that you have in your pockets?"

Fritz pulled it all out, two ashtrays, one napkin, and a set of silverware. He just smiled and said, "You know, this is the first time in my life that I've ever done anything like this."

Later, I called the owner and apologized, and told him about Fritz's disease. He was very understanding. When it had occurred, I was so embarrassed that I wanted to cry. When we returned to our car, I asked him why he had done that. He said, "That was my bonus for all the business that we've given them over the years." At this point, lecturing him seemed futile.

To my knowledge, there was only one other time he was caught shoplifting. That was at the supermarket. I was afraid to leave him in the car, so I sent him in for just one carton of milk. After a while, he came out with the manager following close behind him. The manager was hollering something at Fritz. He got into the car, banged the door shut, and looking very mean said, "Let's get the hell out of here, and I don't want to ever come to this damned store again." He would not tell me what had happened inside the store, and we drove home in silence. I can only guess, that on this day, Fritz felt he was due another bonus.

Fritz became angered if I called an electrician or plumber. It was rather sad, because he had always fixed everything. Now, he could not really fix anything, and more important than that, it was not safe for him to attempt any repairs. For a year or so, absolutely nothing got repaired, unless it was an emergency.

Sometimes he would insist upon helping the repairman, but that always resulted in an argument, since Fritz's way of doing something was the *only* way. He would throw down his wrench or screwdriver and disappear upstairs. After the repairman left, he would give me holy hell. It just crushed my spirit. How do you tell a man that he is not able to fix anything anymore?

Then he started stealing the repairmen's tools. They never saw him. Sometimes, I would find these tools months later, even years later.

Long after Fritz had left home, our San Antonio friends told me that on our last visit in 1988, there had been something missing from their home. It was a pair of two small antique Dresden porcelain roses. They had no doubt that Fritz had taken them, but they didn't want to worry me. Ray had a pair of Dresden candlesticks and three Dresden roses. Ray said, "I'm surprised he didn't take the candlesticks. He knew good stuff." I've never recovered the roses.

When Fritz was on the front courtyard, he struck up conversations with anyone who came walking by. Often, the street people asked him for money, and he liked to give it to them. I kept a supply of five-dollar bills. Fritz would relate to me many of the stories people told him. According to Fritz, there were many of them with Ph.d.s. There were some with two Ph.d.s. One Saturday, one of Fritz's friends came by and asked for money. Fritz came inside to get some money. I was cooking a big pot of chili. Fritz said this guy hadn't eaten for two days, so I fixed him a big bowl of chili and a drink. Fritz took it to him, and returned for some crackers. When Fritz returned with the crackers, his friend was gone, and Iris was just finishing the chili.

For the last three years, I became Fritz's occupational therapist. He would be working on a project and just couldn't make it work. He would say, "I can't do anything anymore."

I would lie, and say, "That's simply not true and you know it." I would work with him on projects, saying things like, "Oh, I know what you're going to do. You're going to put that washer on there." We worked for hours and hours together, and I would let him think he had done it all. It was very frustrating, because usually I could have done it in half the time, or less. I remember one day, it took the entire day to wire one lamp, and I almost tore my hair out . I knew how important it was that he feel he was still useful.

The Chow Dog

We were whiling away the autumn afternoon in the big blue antique rockers on our front porch. It was pleasant . . . just being lazy and listening to the sounds of the season. Gusts of wind blew the big crunchy sycamore leaves, and swirled them around the courtyard. I liked the rustling sound they made as they skipped along the brick. Iris was sleeping between us. After a while the telephone rang, and I left to answer it.

In about two minutes I could hear Fritz hollering, "Liz, get out here . . . help me . . . Liz!" and at first glance I couldn't really tell what was going on . . . Fritz was in the middle of the street with two balls of fast-moving fur, a black one and a red one. There was a lot of activity. He screamed at me, "Come here and help me tear these two apart. Iris is hung up with this damned Chow dog."

I said, "No, get away from them! That Chow is going to bite you!" By this time, I was in the middle of the street, too . . . and screaming at Fritz. I didn't think it was possible, and I don't know how he did it (but I'm sure those big hands certainly helped). Not only did he pull those dogs apart . . . he gave the red Chow two large swift kicks in the ass.

As we returned to our rockers, Fritz said, "Now Iris, don't you ever go messing around with those street dogs again."

The Scavengers

Although I do admit to being more than a bit of a scavenger, I met my match when I met Fritz. Fortunately, we had a Mercedes station wagon, that we purchased after our big yellow truck was stolen. We were always hauling something. We went to estate and garage sales, auctions, and picked up things off the curbs.

As Fritz's disease progressed, the trash put out to the street became more and more attractive to him. He became less and less discriminating as to what he would rescue. It really got to be ridiculous. The study became his trash pile, and almost everything he picked up, he would say, "I can fix that." He had an uncanny way of spotting a piece of trash a block away. He picked up all sorts of building materials, used five-gallon paint cans and many other pieces of trash. He picked up old clothes, shoes, discarded radios and electronic equipment, termite-eaten lumber, broken pieces of glass, pieces of sheetrock and hundreds of plastic flower pots.

I can't begin to tell you the assortment of trash we hauled home. One time he picked up a broken-down baby buggy, which was missing a wheel. Sometimes, we would fill up the station wagon and return for a second trip. When the study was almost filled to the ceiling, he started stashing it outside on the north side of our house. My children began to refer to it as Fritz's alley. One of the worst specimens he brought home was a foul-smelling old mattress. It just sickened me when he brought it inside the house. We had a bit of a heated discussion about that, but I lost.

About a week later, while he was at Rotary Club, I paid someone to haul it off. He never missed it. The lumber with the termites, which he stashed in his alley, turned out to be a real hazard. The termites got into our fence and house, and caused several thousand dollars worth of damage. Of course, neither of us had noticed the termites.

The more Fritz's disease progressed, the more rubbish we hauled home. At one point I suggested he wear gloves. He looked at me like I was out of my mind. Doing my errands presented a logistical problem. I had to arrange them so that my route didn't take me through an area where it was trash pick up day.

Of course, I didn't seek out trash piles, but when Fritz said, "STOP, I see something I want," . . . how could I deny him these pleasures? I would even help him load the trash, but I carried my gloves to use for just such occasions. I would pray that none of our friends would see me perusing in the refuse. I would reminisce about his junk pile down the street from us, and remember the very first time he proudly showed it to me, and how I thought he was so wonderful, and so down to earth. I didn't know that it could get so out of control.

It seemed that Fritz was now a caricature of his original self. When I would see the delight that registered on his face when we came upon a junk pile, it reminded me of a kid in a candy store. How on earth could I pass it by? I only thought, this is what it meant, when on our wedding day I promised, "for better or for worse." This had to be it.

Rabbits in The Grass, Nuts, Screws, Bolts And Forty-Seven Trolls

One of our favorite outings was to visit Teas Nursery. It is like one enormous garden, and when the roses are in bloom, it is divine. Sometimes we would just go there and sit on a garden bench. One day as we walked through the nursery, Fritz pointed to a wall vase and said, "Sweetheart, do you like that?"

I told him yes, that I thought it was very pretty.

About a week later, the same large terra cotta wall vase appeared in Fritz's study with his other collections.

On another occasion, six large cans of tuna fish appeared in our pantry. Never once, did I ever see Fritz take anything, and I thought that I watched him like a hawk. Like Pat said, "He's got the fastest hands in the west."

We bought truffles from friends of ours, who owned a chocolate store on Post Oak Boulevard, close to The Galleria. About a week after we had been there, Fritz said, "Sweetheart, I have a present for you." The present was two chocolate Easter rabbits. When I asked him where he had gotten them, he said, "I just went outside, and there they were, just as big as life, sitting in the grass."

Not until he had left home, and I had cleaned out his collections, did I realize the full extent of his shoplifting. There was a Breitling stopwatch, made in Switzerland, from Best and Co., three stainless steel dental tools, numerous small American flags, forty-seven trolls, thirty pieces of flatware, three silk ties from Neiman-Marcus, an assortment of salt and pepper shakers and thirty-five ash trays. There were many items taken from our local hardware store, including nails, screws, bolts, batteries, an assortment of small tools, a calculator and many other items that I didn't recognize. All of his loot was from places that we frequented on a regular basis, and all of the items had the price tags still on them. How could he have gotten away with all this stuff?

We developed several serious leaks on the ceilings of our living room and bathroom. They were bad enough that we had to put buckets under them when it rained. My son-in-law climbed onto our roof, found the leaks, and determined that we needed a new roof.

Fritz was irate with me. He thought that he should have been the one to climb onto the roof, three stories up. For a month or so, every time Charles came over, he would say, "Tell me, what is it that I'm mad at Charles for?"

The next day I called Sears to come out to give us a bid on a new roof. It took a month before I could get Sears to come give us a bid. There was a reason for that. It was the fourth time Sears had not kept an appointment. I was pretty upset. I called and relayed the entire story to a supervisor, while Fritz sat very quietly and innocently at the table with me. The man said he would investigate and then call me back.

In twenty minutes he called back to say, "Mrs. Becker, today was the fourth time we've sent out a contractor. I guess it's your husband who always met them at your gate. He told all of them that he didn't need a roofer, that he was going to do it himself, and that he could do anything."

I asked Fritz why he had sent the roofers away. He replied, "I didn't know we had a leaky roof, and I don't remember sending anyone away. It's just as well I sent them away, because I'm not going to be paying someone for something I can do myself. It's too hot out there this afternoon, but first thing in the morning, I'm going to be up there laying that roof." There was nothing I could say, and nothing I really wanted to say.

I arranged with Sears to come on three different occasions when Fritz was away bowling. Finally, the roof was completed.

URBAN RENEWAL

During 1986 and 1987, Fritz's activities became more and more dangerous. It was pure Hades for me. He had never liked the looks of the run-down house across the street, where the Mexican family lived. In his study he kept a can of Varsol, that he used for many different things. It was extremely flammable.

Much to my horror, one day I caught Fritz crossing the street with the black dog, a large box of kitchen matches, and the can of Varsol. We stood in the street and argued about it for a couple of minutes. He said it made everything in the neighborhood look bad, and that he had intended for years to burn it down. He said that he had really wanted to do it at night, but he didn't want to hurt anyone. His reasoning was that during the daytime the parents were at work and the children were in school, so this would be his perfect opportunity.

Several blocks down the street I saw a police car coming toward us. I didn't have to continue my pleadings, for Fritz quickly retreated into our house, waving to the officer as he passed by.

That was not to be his last attempt to burn down that house. Three more times he set out with the matches and the can of Varsol. It was unnerving for Pat and me, but we always managed to foil his plans.

Finally, I got rid of the can of Varsol and hid the matches. For months afterward, every night in bed, (when he was apparently planning the next day's activities) Fritz would say, "Sweetheart, you know I can't find my Varsol anywhere. Will you remind me first thing in the morning to go buy some more?"

I would say, "Yes, we'll go buy some, first thing in the morning." Always, in the morning, the Varsol would be long forgotten.

There was a railroad track that occasionally we had to cross. It was the location of several very frightening scenes. A train was coming. The barricades were down and the red lights were flashing. We were the first car in line. When the train was about two-hundred feet away, Fritz began hollering at me to go under the barricades. He opened the door, and with one leg anchored on the street, tried to drag me out of the car. He continued screaming at me and behaving like a maniac until the train passed by.

There were numerous aggravations that continued until Fritz was gone. We had a badly broken glass coffee pot. For six weeks, I put it out with the trash. Every time, he rescued it from the trash, and then stashed it down his alley. Finally, Pat took it home with her and disposed of it with her own trash. That was the only fail-safe technique we could employ to ensure removal of trash that Fritz had taken a liking to.

The poor black dog really suffered with Fritz. He started pinching her ears, pulling her tail, and stepping on her paws. Nevertheless, she stayed right by his side. I thought it remarkable that she didn't bite him. It seemed she sensed that he was ill. Fritz moved so quickly that rarely did Pat or I ever see him do these things. We did hear the black dog yelp.

One day, Fritz stood in the foyer and called me. I had just emerged from the bathtub. Without a stitch on, I came running out, looked over the railing, and there he stood with a street person. As I dashed into the bedroom, I heard Fritz say, "Sweetheart, come down here. I have someone here I know you'll want to meet."

We have a beautiful eighteenth century tall case clock in our foyer. We had never gotten it repaired, because Fritz had always said he was going to fix it. For seven years, he fiddled with it. The last couple of years, he must have taken that clock through the gong cycle twenty to thirty times a day. It had a very primitive and abrasive ding. It drove Pat and I up the wall. Pat said, "You know, I always wanted a grandfather clock, but now, I sure have changed my mind."

Over a period of about three months, I began missing some mail, like bills that I received on a regular basis. Upon investigating, we found that Fritz was putting the mail in the garbage. We finally had to sort through the trash each time, before we put it out to the street.

It was a strange deterioration of his mind. There was no time for trying to explain it. I spent most of my time trying to keep up with him.

Over a period of three or four months, we had maybe fifteen to twenty light bulbs burn out. It was puzzling. Pat suggested that perhaps Fritz might have something to do with it. Indeed, he did. We found that he was unscrewing the bulbs just a tiny bit, just far enough so that they didn't connect.

The last year Fritz was home, was probably the most difficult year of my life. Living with him became very frightening, as well as disruptive. He was a full-time job. He was a very different person than the one I first knew. He had become very paranoid. His personality had changed into something I did not recognize.

To further complicate his ill health, he was diagnosed with diabetes.

For the last six months Pat became so nervous and jumpy that she could hardly sleep at night. In the evenings, upon leaving she would say, "Be careful, and if you should need me in the middle of the night, call me right away. I'll take a cab over."

Fritz tried hard to get Pat to leave. She would not leave because she had become very fond of him. For the last year, every night before she went to bed, Pat would call to check on me. She just wanted to be sure I was safe. She would say, "Mrs. Becker, I know how hard it is for you, but I think the doctors are right. He needs to be in a nursing home." Later, she would tell me that every morning she came to our house, she never knew whether she would find me dead or alive. She also said, "Honey, every night, I pray that he won't kill you tonight."

I would say, "Oh Pat, how could it have come to this?" And, I would cry.

With Fritz's antics Pat always said, "Mrs. Becker, he's working on us." We had a small buffet in the breakfast room, where we kept all of the gardening supplies. One day I came up behind Fritz, where he was standing in front of the open refrigerator. On the counter was a quart of Malathion, a deadly pesticide. The lid was off. Alongside, was an open quart of milk. Fritz was quick to say, "I didn't put that there. Pat must have done that, of course she did."

That was the last time either Pat or I ate anything from open containers in our refrigerator.

It was a long time since Fritz had been rational. Periodically, his doctors would sit me down and tell me what I didn't want to hear, that he was psychotic.

Many times Fritz would steal my keys, and leave the house in the middle of the night, while I was sleeping. I would awaken, and he would not be there beside me. It was terrifying. Always, he hadn't gone far, and I would find him. During the last year, I did not get a decent nights sleep. Three or four times a night, I would awaken to see if he was still there beside me.

The activity that produced the highest level of anxiety in me, was when he started taking knives upstairs to the bedroom at night. I don't even know when it began, because I had never looked in the drawer of his night table. One day I was looking for something in his drawer, and found the butcher knife there. God, that was unnerving. Every night I would check his drawer and there would be a different weapon. He had seven or eight different kinds of knives, and I didn't know where he kept all of them. There were switchblades, Bowie knives, an ice pick, an assortment of screwdrivers and a package of single-edged razor blades.

All of these appeared one at a time, in the drawer of his night table. The worst of all the items was his collection of antique head-hunter knives, that he had brought from Indonesia.

ACUTE ANXIETY ATTACK

One night, I found two of the head-hunter knives in Fritz's night table drawer. As I started to crawl up into our big antique bed, I suddenly became very ill. I got very cold and clammy as I tried again to get into bed. Then I began to shake. I paced around the bedroom, hoping I'd feel better. Once more I tried to get into bed, but I just couldn't seem to get into bed with Fritz. I got sicker and sicker and very weak. I called my daughter, Alison. She and her husband were here in fifteen minutes. Then my son, Travis, came. They took me to the emergency room at St. Joseph's Hospital, downtown. Fritz came along with us. We were there until four o'clock in the morning. The diagnosis was "acute anxiety attack."

Later, my children told me they were afraid that I was going to die. They said I looked dreadful, and that my color was gray.

Another most annoying activity of Fritz's, was putting on a record, and changing the speed setting from 33-1/3 to 45 revolutions per minute. When we inquired about it, he said that the machine was broken. It was a horrible sound, but he would just sit in his chair listening to it for hours, as we wondered how on earth he thought up these bizarre entertainments.

His quietest, and most harmless activity, was picking little specks off of the navy blue carpeting on the stairs. The other quiet time obsession was tearing apart the toilet tissue. Every time we got a new roll of tissue he tore apart every little square, making a neat pile, until it was finished. He spent hours doing these things, and Pat and I were always happy when he took to the stairs, or started his work on the toilet tissue. We knew that for several hours, we would be able to get some work done.

Because I could never take him shopping with me, I would leave him with Pat. She was extremely good with him. Sometimes I would ask her to see to it that Fritz had a bath and was dressed before I returned home. I would then take him to some selected places where I wouldn't be in mortal fear of being arrested for shoplifting. She was much better at getting him to bathe than I was. She was good at devising schemes to get him to cooperate. For instance, she told him that only old men didn't take baths. That worked for quite some time. During the last year, Fritz had absolutely refused to bathe.

On one occasion, I returned home to find Pat in a state of shock. She had told him to go upstairs and take a bath. When she went to check on him, he was sitting in the bathtub fully dressed in his World War II khakis, in a tub full of water. Floating in the water, were pieces of feces. He absolutely refused to move. He sat there until the water got cold, and then he got out of the tub. Pat was there to take charge of the situation, and she gave him holy hell. He just looked mean , not comprehending what all the fuss was about.

"Where Is My Shaving Cream?"

Another day, when Pat was preparing him for an outing, Fritz hollered to her from the upstairs hall, "Pat, Pat, come here right away." Pat hurried to the foyer, looked up and there was Fritz, buck nude, leaning over the railing. He had shaving cream all over his face, and was holding the shaving cream can in his hand. He said, "Pat, where is my shaving cream?"

Very calmly Pat said, "Mr. Becker, the shaving cream is in your hand, and on your face. Now, get in the bathroom and finish shaving." Pat said that she knew from the look on his face that he had staged the incident to shock her. Indeed, he had, but she never let him know that she knew all of his tricks.

Pat and I were never able to figure out how, with his distorted mind, he was able to devise the most complicated booby traps. It was as if there had been a quake inside his brain, and when the layers of memory came back together again, most of the synapses just didn't fit. He built some ingenious booby traps. He set them up in the big armoire in the study, in the refrigerator, in the chef's pantry and in the armoire in our bedroom. It usually took him about an hour to set a perfect trap. He built them with boxes, jars of nails, and just about anything that was handy. They were well-engineered projects, that always produced sound effects. Sometimes, he would use twine to make them work. When the unsuspecting victim opened the door, everything would come crashing down. In the refrigerator and pantry, he devised an elaborate method of stacking the cans, bottles and jars. When the door was opened, everything fell out onto the floor.

Fritz became very testy, and was continually setting up situations to pick a fight with me. He always seemed happy about planting flowers. He could still dig a hole and then plant a flower, but two minutes later he would rip the plant out of the ground. He was so fast, that I usually didn't see him do it. He would blame Iris. After a while, it just wasn't worth it.

One sunny day I was working in the garden. Fritz was sitting on the terrace looking at a book. He liked to look at National Geographic nature books. He left, saying he was going to use the bathroom. After several minutes, from somewhere above, I heard him say, "Hey, Sweetheart!" He was on the third floor south deck, which had no balustrades.

God, he was right close to the edge, urinating. The black dog was standing alongside him. I was terrified, and went outside and calmly pleaded for him to come down. I went into the house, fixed a coke, and prayed to St. Jude for his safety. In about ten minutes he came down. Later, after he had repeated this scene several more times, I had to put locks on the attic doors.

In the guest bedroom there was a large antique armoire that was full of antique linens. There were crocheted and embroidered tablecloths, counterpanes, napkins, and beautiful linen pillow shams with crocheted lace. One day, I opened the armoire to look for a tablecloth. There, I found the most demoralizing sight. On top of every stack of linens, there was a piece that had been cut. There were circles and squares very carefully cut out of about twenty-five pieces. I knew Fritz was a very sick man, but this made me extremely angry. I found it extremely hard to forgive him.

Pat and I began to smell a faint odor of urine in the foyer, but we couldn't find the source. As the weeks went by, the smell became more pungent. Then, one day Pat discovered an amazing thing. Fritz was urinating on the carpeting as he climbed the stairs. She gave him holy hell, telling him that he knew where the toilet was, and, "put that thing away and go up to the bathroom." He did just that, but only temporarily. Hence, Pat had to shampoo the carpeting at least twice a week.

One weekend, when the Italian light show was in Houston, we invited Pat to join us, and offered to take her home after the show. Fritz was about to get into the car when he said he needed to go back inside to use the bathroom. He was gone six to eight minutes, which was longer than we thought he needed to take care of his business. All of us thoroughly enjoyed the light show. It was spectacular.

I was stunned when we returned home. All of my shoes were in a pile on our bedroom floor, and my closet was in complete disarray. Many of my clothes had been moved out of order. Some of them were on the floor. There was scouring powder sprinkled in both bathtubs. He had engineered some sort of structure on the lid of the toilet seat, using large art books from our bedroom, a large Kleenex box, some pictures from my dresser, a can of scouring powder and a bottle of bleach. Lord, what a creation.

There was another surprise for me. As I pulled back the covers to get into bed, heavens, there was dog hair and dirt all over my side of the bed, and on my pillow. Apparently, he had shaken the dog's rug onto my side of the bed. It was difficult to believe that in such a short period of time, he was able to accomplish so much.

The last Christmas Fritz spent at home was during 1986. His son and family, including Fritz's only three grandchildren, paid their regular brief visit on Christmas day. I talked to his son about how very ill his father was, and asked if he would bring the children by to visit him. He promised he would, and that was the last time he was ever in our house.

As Fritz's mind became more disturbed, the damages mounted. One day, Pat and I heard a loud noise coming from the powder room. Fritz had put his fist through the wall. On another occasion, Fritz cut the garden hose in five places.

The most aggravating of all of his capers, was the damage he did to our Mercedes. He broke off the antenna, broke off every knob that he could manage, including the control that moved the seat on the passenger side. He tore out a large piece of the interior wall under the dash, and took a key or coin and scraped the exterior paint. For months, he would get into the car and change the setting to "off" on the dome light. It was just an aggravation, because the light didn't come on when the door was opened. Although we had new tires, I had many flats. The repairman suggested that probably someone was letting the air out of my tires, since he couldn't find any damage to them.

Fritz would say, "Look at that. We've got a flat. I'm going to drive down and get some air in that tire." That never happened. I guarded my keys like a hawk.

Always, Fritz had been a very territorial animal. He became enraged when anyone parked in front of our house, most especially when they parked at the end of our sidewalk. My daughter, Alison, experienced thirty-two flat tires over a period of seven years. The service people always found nails in her tires. My son also had countless flat tires. I paid a visit next door, where I was told that many of their guests were having a number of flats, and it had been happening for years.

I suggested to my children that I thought Fritz was putting nails in their tires. In his study he kept some twenty jars of nails. Most of them were large and old and rusty. My children absolutely refused to believe he would do such a thing. It continued for years. One day, I caught him in the act. He placed one large nail in the back of one front tire, with the head propped on the ground. If one backed up, the nail punctured the tire. He arranged another nail on the rear tire, so that if one went forward, the tire was pierced by the nail.

It wasn't until after he had been gone for a year or so, that my children realized they had not had a single flat tire since he had left. It was only then that they would believe that Fritz might have had anything to do with their frequent flat tires.

Fritz derived a great deal of satisfaction from just sitting in his chair in the living room after dark. He would put on the low voltage spotlights, and (as he put it), "just soak up the beauty around me." Many times he would call me in and say, "Sweetheart, come sit on the love seat with me. There's really nothing in the kitchen that you just have to do." His eyes would sparkle, and he exuded a radiance, as he looked about the room, seeing the results of his labors. It made me feel good to see his pleasure. He would say, "Sweetheart, I owe all of this to you."

Candlelight Lament

On one such evening, at Fritz's request, I joined him on the love seat in the living room. He was counting the blessings of his life, and I was at the top of his list. He inquired as to where we had gotten various pieces. Then he said, "Why don't you light the candles?" I did, all fourteen of them.

He continued to congratulate us on our talents and accomplishments. He said that there wasn't anything that we couldn't do, together. He prided himself on his self-reliance and independence. In the candlelit room, in the most sincere and romantic terms, he began to tell me just how much I meant to him. His voice became a monotone, and it was as if he were in a trance. He had a far away look in his eyes, and a diabolical look on his face. He held my hand with a crushing grip. He said he wanted to put some new policies in place.

First and foremost, he wanted to fire Pat. He did not want anyone to come inside our house. We would have complete privacy. The second thing was, there was no reason why we ever needed to leave our house again, because we had everything we needed right here. He went on to say that we would get all of our food delivered. At that point he asked me to get some paper and a pencil. For over an hour, we made a weekly menu and a grocery list. All of these were multiplied by fifty-two. For instance, fifty-two cans of tuna fish, sixty pounds of sugar, etc. When all of this was completed, I inquired as to what we would do about fresh meat and vegetables. He was disappointed when he had to concede to a weekly grocery delivery, but the delivery people would be instructed to leave the groceries on the porch.

After that was settled, I told Fritz that I thought I would go upstairs to bed. He grabbed my arm, sinking his strong big fingers into my flesh, and angrily said, "You don't want to sit here with me. Why?"

I told him that I was tired and wanted to go to bed. Still, with his hand holding my arm, he began to pursue a ridiculous line of conversation. It had to do with my love for him. He was convinced that I did not love him anymore. Through all of this, I kept thinking of the film, "Gaslight," with Ingrid Bergman and Charles Boyer. Suddenly, he let go of me, and hit me hard in the top of my arm.

Our regular routine, when we went up to bed, was that Fritz secured the doors. I went upstairs first, and he followed with the black dog.

I ran into the foyer and started up the stairs. He was right behind me. He broadsided me with his arm, and knocked me down. I managed to get up, and ran up to the landing on the stairs. Looking up at me, with a crazed look on his face, he said, "Sweetheart, are you going to cut my throat?"

I was horrified, and wanted to burst into tears. My blood ran cold. Very calmly, I said, "Of course not, Darling, I love you. Now, why don't you check the doors, and come on upstairs to bed."

We had a large Bible on the piano with oversized print. During the last few months he began reading it. I'd never seen him read the Bible before. Long after he had left home, I was browsing in the Bible and turned to where he had left the book mark. It was marked at the "Ten Commandments." The commandment, "Thou shalt not kill," was underlined.

The Branding Iron

The branding iron was kept behind the kitchen door. It had a block-lettered "B" on the end of it. It was old and rusty.

These nights it was difficult to get a whole nights' sleep. Fritz was up and down, and sometimes in and out of the house.

I awakened in the middle of the night and opened my eyes. Fritz was standing over me, holding the branding iron, with a fiendish look in his eyes. "Sweetheart, let's dance." It was three o'clock in the morning, and I diplomatically declined. With the progression of the disease he had become more and more cantankerous. Not wanting to precipitate a nasty argument, I thought cooperation was in order, and that meant accepting his invitation to dance.

He gallantly helped me down from our bed, and began singing, "It's three o'clock in the morning." Holding me tightly, and still grasping the branding iron, which was behind my back, he waltzed me around the bedroom. As we passed the large Victorian dresser, in the mirror I could see reflected this most ridiculous scene.

We danced to many of his favorite tunes, that he most enthusiastically sang, "Ain't she sweet? See her coming down the street, and I tell you very confidentially, ain't she nice? Look her over once or twice," etc. Then there was, "I can't give you anything but love, Baby," and "Mean to me. Why must you be mean to me?" Then the dancing turned to marching to, "The Saints Go Marching In." Things got louder and livelier, and his fervor peaked.

It seemed to go on forever. We marched all around, up and down, on all three floors to the strains of "Saints," and "The Battle Hymn of the Republic." All the while Fritz brandished his monogrammed branding iron. We were breathless. On one trip down he stopped at the record machine and put on "Beethoven's Military Music," and we continued.

On the fourth trip downstairs, he stopped at the refrigerator. What a welcome diversion, Blue Bell Ice cream. Decisions came to him with much difficulty these days. Thank God for vanilla, and only vanilla. He prepared our two festive green bowls heaping full, and we returned to our boudoir. While his back was turned, I hid the branding iron in the fireplace.

His mood gradually became more subdued, as he methodically fed me the ice cream, "one for you and one for me, one for you and one for me." After a while I felt a little bit sick, and just before I fell asleep, I remember thinking that I wasn't sure if "Battle Hymn of the Republic" was still my favorite song.

Years before, we had become friends with a black antique dealer named Le Roy. He and Fritz got along famously. During the last year, when we visited his shop, we couldn't keep Fritz out of his trash cans. They were outside at the rear of his property.

Le Roy would say, "Mrs. Becker, just let him be. He's having fun. Take him home and dip him."

Le Roy was one of a number of friends who were very concerned about Fritz living at home. He knew how bad he had gotten, and he feared for my safety. He felt that he should be in a nursing home. One day, while Fritz was out back going through the trash cans, Le Roy said, "Mrs. Becker, sometimes I drive by your house around midnight. I look up at the balcony doors to your bedroom, and think, God, I hope Mr. Becker doesn't wake up in the middle of the night, and choke you to death with those big hands."

I said, "Don't you think I haven't thought of it." Then, I thought of the very first time I met Fritz, and how I was so taken with his incredible hands.

In memory of our mothers, we had planted a pair of tall, watermelon-red crape myrtle trees in front of our house. They were about thirty feet tall. Fritz tore off a huge branch from his mother's tree. I prefer to think that he had forgotten that the tree had been planted for his mother.

Lizzy Borden

It was a Saturday morning. Pat was working in the kitchen and I was in the breakfast room taking care of some business. Fritz was in the study, doing, we didn't know what, but we thought there was a good possibility that he was building another trap. Fortunately, we always expected the unexpected. Fritz appeared in the doorway, with his hatchet and his sharpening tool. After a few minutes, I suggested that he put the hatchet away. He ignored me. He set about sharpening the hatchet. It was very unnerving. He paced about the kitchen and breakfast room sharpening his hatchet for the entire day. I could only think of "The Legend of Lizzy Borden." He sat down once, with me, at the breakfast room table for about a half hour, sharpening his hatchet all the while.

He looked up at the ceiling fan, which was turned on, and said, "Look, look, look at the geese flying around." Pat said it was the longest day she had ever spent here.

Fritz was watching a baseball game one afternoon, when I left to do some errands. When I returned several hours later, Pat said that every ten minutes he had asked where I was. Every time he asked, he said, "You know Pat, I think she's run off with Le Roy."

For the last three years, several times a week, just before we went to sleep, Fritz would say, "Now, first thing in the morning I'm going to crawl under the house and put in a water line so we can have a faucet on the south side. Would you like that?"

I would say, "Yes, that would be a good thing to do." I would think, "Isn't it marvelous that he still looks forward to the next day." As diseased as his mind was, I found it phenomenal that he could still have that good feeling that there was a job in the morning that he felt he could do. It didn't make a difference that he really was not capable of doing the job. What was important was that he thought he could do it. To have something to look forward to, I believe, is essential for a happy life. Of course, I knew that in the morning, he would have forgotten about the faucet.

During the last three months he lived at home, he became obsessed with his project in the attic. That was laying down the pre-World War II oak flooring that he had collected. I was amazed that he even remembered how to do it. He had installed the flooring in eight of our rooms seven years ago. He had to use his power table saw to cut the wood. I didn't think he should be doing that and discussed it with him. He said that I should check with his doctor, and he would abide by the doctor's decision. To my astonishment, the doctor said it was all right. It was quite a job. The floor measured about fifteen by thirty feet, and he pounded the hell out of those nails. Most of the time, he would not take breaks, even for lunch. I brought his lunch up to him. The black dog stayed right with him, and every time I heard the noise of the saw, I hoped that he still had all of his fingers.

That last visit to his doctors in the medical center, before he left home, was memorable. First, the doctor talked to me in private. I told him some of the very hostile things he had done. During every appointment in the last two years, he had recommended that I place Fritz in a nursing home. He would say, "Mrs. Becker, what are you waiting for?" I would say, "I plan to take care of him as long as I am physically and mentally able." Always, I had felt that I could do almost anything. Today, I didn't feel nearly as sure that I was able to do this much longer. I told him so.

He said, "Mrs. Becker, you have kept him years more than most people would have. You look as if you've lost weight. You look depressed. Now, promise me that you will give serious consideration to placing him in a home. I know it's hard for you to let go."

I swallowed a huge lump in my throat, brushed away the tears, and said, "I'll think it over."

After we talked, we joined Fritz and four other resident psychiatrists. All of us sat around a table and the doctors asked Fritz questions, his name, where he lived, and then the sixty-four-dollar question, "Mr. Becker, what was your career? What did you do for a living?"

With great dignity, Fritz replied, "I was Field Chief of the C.I.A. for Texas and New Mexico for twenty-four years." The doctors looked at each other very skeptically, as if to say, "Mr. Becker, do you really expect us to believe that?" Then one of them said, "Mr. Becker, you said the C.I.A., tell us about that."

I looked around the table, to see all of those psychiatrists stroking their chins. After a few minutes of questioning, I couldn't stand to see it continue. I interrupted, telling them that yes, he had indeed been Field Chief of the C.I.A. for Texas and New Mexico for twenty-four years. They did look surprised, and then all of the doctors congratulated him. Fritz beamed, and looked proud and pleased. I shared his joy.

After we returned home, night and day, the doctor's strong recommendation took over my thinking. I felt as if I was about to plunge into a tank of acid, and couldn't make the decision as to when I would do it. I couldn't bear the thought of living without him. Furthermore, I had never lived alone, ever. The doctor's words came to me, "You have nothing to feel guilty about." I did feel guilty. I felt consumed with guilt. After about four weeks of indecision and many more tears, I decided that if I loved him, I must place him in a nursing home. I would deal with my emotions later.

Shortly after I had made that agonizing decision, and was having a great deal of trouble living with it, Pat called out to me in a very distressed and urgent voice. I was in the guest bedroom marking Fritz's clothes to take with him to the home. She was across the hall in the guest bathroom. She said, "Look, you need to come see this."

There were two old boxes, one about ten by fourteen inches, and the other a great deal smaller. The smaller box was a very dark green, and it was a hard cardboard. Inside it, were two of the old glass medical syringes, like the kind used during the fifties. Also, in the box were three bottles of medication, with old yellowed labels on them. They were both sealed, and were from the Avalon Drug Co., close to where Fritz used to live in River Oaks during the fifties. They were labeled, but without a date. They had Fritz's name on them. One was atropine, another was paregoric, and the other epinephrine.

In the larger box were surgeon's gloves. Pat said that this was the first time she had looked in the box, but that during the last year, he had moved them about four times. They were first in the attic, then in his desk, and then in the study. They had just appeared in the bathroom that very day. She said that they were always left out in plain view, and she couldn't believe that I had never seen them.

I felt as if I were going to faint. I began to tremble, and I lay down on the floor. Instantly I remembered the time he had told me how he had very carefully planned to kill his retarded son, who was then a baby. God!

Thank God, that Pat was there to hug me. After I felt I could navigate on my own, I took a long and leisurely ride, alone, in Memorial Park. As I was leaving, I noticed that Fritz was sitting in his chair reading the Bible. Right then and there, I thanked God that his doctor had helped me make the right decision. I never again questioned that decision.

I did lots of research and visited many nursing homes. The decision was made to place him in a personal care home. It was very different than a nursing home. There were only eight patients, and it was more like a real home. It was in the Tanglewood area back in the woods and surrounded by tall trees. It was a painful procedure, but I put together a photo album for him, with pictures taken on our trips, and pictures of our families. I packed up many of his favorite things, including his ukulele, his Indonesian wood carvings, and his favorite nature books. I felt as if I were preparing a child for boarding school.

The doctor suggested that it would probably be better if we did not tell him ahead of time, because of his history of hostility. The night before we took him, as we were lying in bed that night Fritz said, "Sweetheart, first thing in the morning, remind me to crawl under the house and start laying the pipe, so we can have a faucet on the south side." In the darkness, I turned way over to the edge of my side of the bed, and silently cried myself to sleep.

My son and my son-in-law accompanied Fritz and me to the home. We stayed with him for about three hours, getting him settled. For both of us, parting was pure hell. He ran after me, screaming, and three big black women had to hold him. Without a doubt, it was the hardest, and most traumatic event of my life. I sobbed most of the way home, and as I talked about

Fritz, I kept calling him "Tom," my first husband's name. I've never been able to figure that one out. My daughter spent the night with me.

Around three o' clock in the morning, I went downstairs for a glass of milk. As I switched on the light, at the back door, standing with its nose pressed against the glass, was a huge raccoon. I had never seen a raccoon. My first thought was that I was beginning to lose my mind. I didn't really get much sleep that night.

The next day, Fritz's secretary from the C.I.A.office called me. He had called her to enlist her aid in getting him returned home. It was amazing that after more than ten years he was able to remember his old office phone number. She said he was very distraught. He also called other friends. He told them that I was having an affair with another man, and that was the reason I wanted him out of the picture. Of course, none of them believed him. It was all very heartbreaking for me.

We had taken him to the home on November 13th. A couple of weeks later was Thanksgiving. I visited him every day the first couple of weeks. That was tough. Every day, as I left, there was a bad scene. While shouting, he would run after me to the car, and again and again they would have to hold him. For me, a trip to visit him, was like going to hell and back.

My daughter, Katie, arrived from Philadelphia on Thanksgiving day. She was very disturbed with me for putting Fritz in the home. She was angry. Of course, she had no idea of the extent of deterioration of Fritz's mind that had occurred since she had seen him a year ago.

After the hugs and kisses, Fritz and Katie sat down on the couch to visit. Immediately, Katie burst into uncontrollable tears. I was really upset with her. I left the room, and when I returned they were engaged in conversation. Later, I learned that she had agreed with Fritz that she would help him get returned home. She did not think he belonged there. It wasn't until much later that she realized why he could not live at home. She only thought that I had done a heartless and terrible thing by putting him in the home.

Shortly thereafter, Katie had reason to give some serious thought to my point of view regarding Fritz being in the home. June, the jovial, big afro-american manager of the home told me that they were having a lot of trouble with Fritz. He was stealing all sorts of things, mainly from other patients. He had quite a number of built-in drawers beside his bed where he stashed his stolen goods. June said she always knew where to look if something were missing.

Clearly, there was one thing that disturbed June. Every day Fritz would steal her butcher knife from the kitchen. She would have to go looking through all of his drawers, because he would never admit to taking the knife. One day her butcher knife was missing again. She approached Fritz, but he immediately denied having the knife. She went through all of his drawers, and finally found it. She said, "Fritz, please don't take my knife again. I need this knife every day to fix your dinner. Now, Fritz, what do you need a butcher knife for?" After a bit, he replied, "I might have to eliminate my children."

God, I knew that he did not like, or want anything to do with his children, but I hadn't any notion that the hate was so deep-seated. He very often referred to his children as "a bunch of reprobates." I never understood why, but there must have been a lot of things in his past that contributed to his attitude. Just before I took him to the home, Pat said to him, "Mr. Becker, why do you always call your kids reprobates? What is a reprobate?"

He told her that a reprobate was a "bad, no-count person."

The holiday season of 1987 was just miserable for me. I didn't put up a Christmas tree, and didn't attend a single party. I only wanted the holidays to be over, so that I could attempt to straighten out my life.

I had believed that life would be considerably easier with Fritz gone, but that wasn't soon to happen. Every few days, when I visited him, it was like a large wound being ripped open, before it had a chance to heal. I would have to drive home, with the tears streaming down my face.

At home I seemed to get lost. There was an enormous void in my life. Our house was large, twelve rooms in all, and everywhere around me, I could see the results of Fritz's labors. For about a month, the black dog cried. She went from room to room whimpering, and looking for Fritz. Then, she would stand at the attic door, crying. This is where, for the last couple of months, she had spent so much time with him, while he had pounded down the hardwood flooring. She had never left his side.

Now, she quickly attached herself to me, and now I take her almost everywhere. After all, who would attempt a car-jacking with a big Black Labrador in the front seat?

Right around Christmas, I didn't think that things could get much worse, but they did. Fritz's daughter, Brenda, from California, arrived in town. She made a nasty scene at the home in front of Fritz. She was completely out of control; with dancing eyes, she screamed at me. What she wanted was a copy of Fritz's will. I felt so bad for him. I told her to ask him what he would like to do about the matter. He denied her a copy of his will, and she was livid.

The next day he said, "I'll be glad when she goes back to wherever-the-hell she came from."

THE ALAMO

I don't know why I felt so compelled to take that final trip to San Antonio. Perhaps it was pure desperation at trying to hold onto our love affair. There were always people around at the home, and I never felt we had any privacy. Our trips had always been so full of enchantment. I guess I was grasping at anything that I thought might restore some of those vital feelings that seemed to be slipping away. San Antonio, the birthplace of Fritz's ancestors, and a familiar place to him, seemed the right choice.

The two-hundred-mile trip was uneventful. Midway we stopped for lunch at Frank's, a familiar rest stop between Houston and San Antonio. I didn't have to worry about Fritz damaging the car's interior on the trip. He had just about destroyed everything he could get his hands on, inside the car, during the last year.

We checked into the nineteenth century Menger Hotel, where Fritz's aunt gave many fancy parties during the twenties and thirties. It is next door to the Alamo.

After freshening up, and a little rest, we went down to the Riverwalk. We browsed in some of the shops and stopped at a little cafe, for some coffee. We had a wonderful Mexican dinner, and retired early to our hotel room.

On Saturday morning we had breakfast sent up. I remember wishing that things were the way they used to be.

After breakfast we took a ride, and I showed Fritz where his grandparent's home used to be. Of course, he didn't remember. We returned to the hotel for a nice lunch. Then we strolled over to the Alamo. I looked at Fritz and couldn't help thinking how great he looked in his gray flannel pants, navy blue cashmere blazer, blue Oxford cloth button down collar shirt, and a red raw silk tie. He certainly was a handsome devil.

There was not a hint that there was anything wrong with him, at least right then. He paused, tweaked my cheek, and said, "Sweatheart, you're a beautiful woman."

We walked around the Alamo, and its grounds, for several hours. It was the end of January, and a bit chilly, so we decided to leave. As we were leaving, I noticed Fritz stuffing something into his pockets. Oh yes, it was the Christmas lights that the workers were taking down. I pleaded with him to put them down, but my words fell on deaf ears. Oh God, he just kept stuffing them in all of his pockets. I told him they were old and useless, that he didn't need them, and that he would get arrested. He continued to go about his business of winding up the long strings of lights and filling up his pockets.

Finally we left, and walked through the hotel lobby and into the elevator with wires and lights hanging out of the bulging pockets of Fritz's cashmere coat. I noticed a few puzzled glances in the elevator.

Back in the hotel room, Fritz inspected his treasures, untangled them, plugged them into the socket to test them, and then very carefully hung them on a coat hanger. Then we lay down on the bed for a little rest. After I was sure that Fritz was asleep, I took the strings of lights down to the front desk and without explanation, asked if they would take them next door to the Alamo. They looked as if they thought it a curious request, but said, "No problem."

When Fritz awakened, we dressed and went back down to the Riverwalk for dinner. He stooped to pick up a lucky penny, and presented it to me. As for his precious Christmas lights, Fritz never mentioned them again.

The next day was "Super Bowl Sunday." Several good friends, who lived in San Antonio, were to come to our room to watch the game. They were bringing beer and sandwiches. Less than an hour before they were due to arrive, I went into the bathroom to freshen up. Fritz was waiting to take a shower. When I emerged from the bathroom, Fritz was nowhere to be found. I was terrified. I noticed the ice bucket was missing, so I ran down the hall to the ice machine. There was no one in sight. Not knowing what else to do, I took the elevator to the lobby. He wasn't there, either. I returned to our room, hoping to find him there. He was not there, and I began to tremble. Before my anxieties overcame me, I dashed to the elevator and returned to the lobby.

The elevator doors slowly opened, and lo and behold, directly across, in the opposite elevator, stood Fritz, clutching the ice bucket. He was dressed only in his boxer underwear. Up walked our friends. Ray could see that Fritz didn't recognize him, and said, "Fritz, I'm Ray. Remember me, Ray ?"

Fritz replied, "I'm Fritz Becker, and I'm from Houston, Texas, but I don't exactly know where I am right now, but I think I'm at The Holiday Inn, outside Houston.

Ray whispered to me, "What is Fritz doing in the lobby without his clothes?" Ray, very alertly gave our strange looking party a polite shove into the elevator, and we were on our way up. As I glanced across at Fritz, I could see that he looked somewhat confused. He said, "Liz, what did you do with my coat?" I thought, "As sad as it is, I *do* know that this is our last trip." This had been a mistake. Indeed, this was certainly an unforgettable "Super Bowl Sunday."

After the San Antonio trip, I didn't feel especially comfortable taking Fritz out in the car, but it was something he really enjoyed, so I took that risk. God knows, taking risks seemed to be a way of life for me. I did place some restrictions on our travel... no long trips, no travel on the freeways, and give a wide berth to railroad tracks.

The Woodpecker

One balmy April day, I stopped at Otto's Barbecue for some drinks and barbecue, and then picked up Fritz. It was only about a mile from the home to the arboretum in Memorial Park. We parked our car and walked deep into the woods, to our familiar spot. We spread out our blanket and lay down. Fritz kissed me, and held me very close for a long time. It just seemed right that we should make love, and so we did. The woods were still and quiet, except for the incessant sound of a woodpecker, high in the tree above us. For a long time afterward, every time we went out in the car, Fritz said, "Are we going to the woods?"

For our wedding anniversary, in May, we always went to Tony's for dinner, and so this year we had our usual lovely dinner there. Sadly, it wasn't the same. It had become increasingly more difficult to have a conversation with Fritz. He wasn't able to read any more, and what he saw on television, he didn't remember. I would tell myself, "He still has that infectious grin. He still has that sparkle in his eyes that makes me feel so good. And I still love the way he offers me his arm as we walk down the street. So, don't think of all the things he can't do. You can't change that. Look for the things he *can* do. Those things are there.

At Tony's, we sat in the rear on a newly upholstered bench. As we were preparing to leave, Tony brought us a bottle of wine for our anniversary. As we stood up, I looked down at where Fritz had been sitting, and there was a large puddle of urine on the new Scalamandre silk bench. I looked at Fritz, and he looked a little confused. I just felt sad for him. I desperately wanted to change things, a lot of things. I found Tony and apologized, and explained Fritz's condition. He was very gracious, and made me feel like it was not such an unusual happening.

At the home Fritz resumed his habit of urinating here and there, namely in clothes drawers beside his bed. When I opened a drawer, well, the smell was most disagreeable. Then Fritz started leaving little nocturnal gifts for the management, on the kitchen counter. They took the form of a large mound of feces in a cereal bowl, left anonymously. Of course, they knew just who to thank.

Since Fritz had become diabetic, I had to find a new place to buy sugar-free truffles. About once a week I would stop at Bering's to buy regular truffles for me, and sugar-free truffles for Fritz. He was always delighted to have a truffle.

As I was leaving the home one night, Fritz looked up at the full moon, and said, "Look, look. What is that?" I told him think real hard to see if he could remember. After a minute he said, "It's a Rousseau moon." I was amazed. On occasion, when there was a beautiful full moon, I used to refer to it as a Rousseau moon, after a painting by Rousseau. Always, after such an incident, I felt very sad. The whole arrangement did not seem right to me. Why should he be living here, and me be living there? How did this ever come about?

The doctor had said that Alzheimer's was a degenerative disease, ending in death, and that there would be a loss of all intellectual functions, that incontinence would occur, and all speech would be lost. There was no cure. I remember thinking at the time, that those were cruel words. Now, it was five years later, and as those words came back to me loud and clear, I realized that there was no kind way to say these things. They were hard, cruel words, *and they were all true.*

During the next five years, I would come to know, first hand, the full significance of the doctor's words. If anything, it would be all much worse than the doctor's words. After all, those were *only* words.

After several years, it became necessary to move Fritz to a regular nursing home. The home was about a half-block off of Westheimer, a very busy street. Fritz's room was next to the exit door. He quickly figured that out, and about ten times a day he escaped. He would run like a bat out of hell, with someone in hot pursuit after him. Fortunately, he never made it to the street. I was there often, checking things out.

One day I came at lunch and found Fritz licking his chops while he was eating a big piece of chocolate cake. I found that he had been on a regular diet for a week, when they had been given doctor's orders for a diabetic diet. After about a month the management requested that we find another home for him. I was told that I was the reason for this, that I was a trouble maker, and was always hanging around.

The new home had a locked Alzheimer's unit that had just opened. For the first six months, a lady named Mabel, took a fancy to Fritz. She wouldn't let another woman near him. When I would visit, I would find them cuddled up on the sofa, holding hands. Fritz would be looking quite pleased. Mabel would ask me what I wanted and I would say, "I'm here to visit with Fritz. He's my husband."

She would throw a fit and holler at me, "He's my husband. He's not your husband." One time she attacked me with her purse. After a while, they would have to take her away. In about six months, Mabel was moved to another home.

Fritz continued to deteriorate both physically and mentally. He now required an insulin shot daily. He was becoming less mobile, and had difficulty in walking. He became much less social, and hardly talked at all. He was totally incontinent.

The last couple of years were just about more than I could bear. He was confined to a wheelchair, and did not appear to recognize anyone. Sometimes I thought he knew me, but I could never be sure. Even something as basic as feeding himself, he could not do. If I arrived at lunch or dinner, I would feed him. I remember, shortly after we were married, Fritz saying to our friends, "I'm taking care of her now, and she's going to take care of me later." As I fed him lunch one day, I thought, "And how did you know that?"

During this time, I decided I needed something to distract me from his impending demise. My church had a program where they served breakfast, on weekdays, to homeless people. This temporarily eased the pain that I faced each day. When one comes face to face with those without homes, and those who are hungry, it changes the direction of one's thinking. I definitely needed a new direction for my thinking.

On Thanksgiving, 1992, my daughter, Katie, came from Philly to visit Fritz. Before we went to visit I tried to give her an overview of his condition, so she would not be shocked. Also, I gave her a stern talking-to about keeping her emotions under control. I told her I didn't want a crying scene like last time.

Fritz had always been very fond of Katie. She adored him, and he spoiled her. It was a good visit. His eyes sparkled, he smiled, and he held her hand tightly. It was the last time I ever heard him talk. Katie's hair was in her face, and with his big hand, he brushed her hair out of her eyes and said, "Hair."

On May twenty-fifth, our fourteenth wedding anniversary, I went for a visit with Fritz. I had spent an extra amount of time primping and dressing. He always had appreciated me looking pretty. As I drove out to see him, I thought of our anniversary and felt very sad. Even though he couldn't talk to me now, I always talked to him, as if he understood. Who knows, maybe he did. This day he had on his Texas A & M baseball cap. Several times he smiled. I asked him, "Are you a Texas Aggie?"

He looked as if he wanted to talk, and then he just grunted. Then for the sixty-four-dollar question, "Do you love me?" He gave a big grunt, I hugged him hard, and that is how we celebrated our fourteenth wedding anniversary.

TRUFFLES

"The soul can split the sky in two,
And let the face of God shine through."

From "Renascence" by Edna St. Vincent Millay

Intermittently, over the past five years, there was something that was giving me a great deal of mental distress. For the past year, as I lay in bed at night, I couldn't seem to dispose of some disturbing thoughts. They had become a burden for me. I kept remembering the night of Fritz's mother's funeral. He had said to me, "Sweetheart, if I should lose my mind, like my mother, I don't want to live. You're a very smart woman, and if you don't know how to carry out my wishes, then you make it your business to find out." Over and over again, his words returned to torment my nights.

One day, during the first week of June, I had an especially bad night of tossing and turning. I recounted Fritz's words after his mother's funeral. I decided to visit Fritz. On the way, I stopped to purchase a truffle for him. He would like that. I walked slowly around the candy counter several times. I don't know why I did that, because I always knew just exactly what I wanted. I wanted a sugar-free truffle and a regular truffle, and I would buy them and be gone. Today, I must have been there for ten minutes. Several times the sales girl said, "May I help you?"

She seemed to speak in a faraway voice. I didn't really know why I was pacing around the counter. It was as if I was in a trance.

I knew what I had to do. I stopped in front of the truffles. They all seemed to be growing larger, and seemed as if they were moving toward me. I couldn't remember how many I needed. I began to tremble, as I purchased one sugar-free truffle and one regular truffle. Actually, my plan had called for two regular truffles.

On the way to the nursing home, the plan took shape. Actually, it was a very simple plan. Fritz was in very poor physical condition, and was a serious diabetic. I would feed him the *regular* truffle. This would send him into a diabetic coma, hastening his death. It occurred to me that I didn't know why I had bought a sugar-free truffle, habit I guess.

It was just after lunch when I arrived at the home. Over the past three months, Fritz had lost seventeen pounds. He sat all by himself in his wheelchair, looking thin and very lonely. I removed the truffle from the bag to begin feeding it to him. Suddenly, there was a bit of a sparkle in his eyes, as he grabbed my hand with a crushing grip. He opened his mouth to bite into the truffle, and I said, "Oh God, no." I dropped the truffle back into the bag and then fed him the sugar-free truffle. On the way home I thought, "He wasn't even aware of it, but he had certainly placed a heavy burden on me."

Several days later, I had a call from the home saying that Fritz was on his way to the hospital. They said that his blood sugar level had risen to over four hundred. He was kept in the hospital until his blood sugar level returned to normal, about a week. I was still plagued by Fritz's words, "You're a very smart woman, and if you don't know how to carry out my wishes, then you make it your business to find out." Oh, if only those words would fade away, but they continued to haunt me.

About a week later, I found myself once again at the truffle store. Again, I paced around the counter. Then, very quietly, I asked for two regular chocolate truffles.

As I drove out to visit Fritz, very deliberately, I expelled all thoughts from my head, and turned up the radio very loud. I arrived at the home, and walked down the long corridor, clutching the tiny bag with the two regular ruffles. Suddenly, I made an unplanned stop at the ladies room. The next thing I was aware of was a loud flushing sound. I looked down, and saw two chocolate truffles swirling and disappearing down the white porcelain commode. I sighed.

The Death of a Lioness

"But O heart! heart! heart!
O the bleeding drops of red,
Where on the deck my Captain lies,
Fallen cold and dead."

From O Captain! My Captain! by Walt Whitman

He lay there, a ghost of the man he'd once been, helpless, pale and frail. Even so, I recognized just a hint of resolve that remained part of his demeanor. He was incontinent and could not talk, but there was still sport in his eyes.

Directly, his food arrived and his eyes did a little dance. There was a bit of a smile. As I fed him dinner, scenes of those very first days, almost twenty years ago, returned. I remembered when I was ill with encephalitis, how he had fed me, how he had taken such very good care of me, and how I had always felt I was being treated like an eggshell. Is this what he meant when he used to say, "I'm taking care of you now, and you're going to take care of me later. Sweetheart, that's quid pro quo, and you know what that means." And, of course I did. Yes, this was quid pro quo. I had the feeling that he knew just what I was thinking. Toward the end I didn't talk much. For his comfort, I tried to remember some of the principles that directed his actions. From the beginning, he had told me, "Sweetheart, I *HATE* small talk."

Early on, and after it had become necessary to place him in a home, seven years ago, I would tell him things I'd done, irritations associated with his absence. All of this pained him. He didn't want to think of me living in our house alone, having to do my own grocery shopping, having to fix my own breakfast, and doing all those things that he felt he should be doing. His powerful desire to take care of me would well up in him and would show itself, and there would be tears in the lioness's eyes. I would have to assume all this phony bravery, that wasn't there. I would have to close the spigot on my tears and say, "Sweetheart Pie, everything is fine, and I'm doing all right." I would look at the lioness, who sorely knew that was a lie, nothing more and nothing less.

After dark, I sat in silence about an hour or so. As he often did, he held my hand with a crushing grip, and with his eyes riveted on mine. He would not let go of my hand. Sometimes, for a bit of comic relief, I would think of that party, when he crashed the Baccarat crystal on the counter, caught the rat, and pinched off its head with his bare hands.

Around eleven o'clock his lids became heavy and moved slowly, open and closed, and then finally closed. A wave of satisfaction showed on his face. He squeezed my hand. Again, we silently plighted our troth to one another.

Shortly thereafter, the big old spotted hand slowly opened, and my hand fell out. I sat in the darkness and listened to the rhythm of his slow respirations. It was rare for me to spend the night, but there was an extra bed. For some reason I wanted to be there, simply that and nothing more. I kissed him on the forehead and lay down on the bed.

At the end of the night, and just before dawn, the wind howled loudly and there were several claps of thunder. It seemed the lightning struck right inside the room, and I was sore afraid. The rain came down in sheets. It was an Edgar Allen Poe night.

I rose from my bed, and switched on the night light. My watch showed five-thirty. Something about the room was not right. Pure terror struck me.

The lioness was not breathing.

With my tears flooding his face, and a large lump in my throat, I flung my body over his. My heart quaked, and I wanted to throw myself into the bayou. I pressed my ear tightly to his chest, and tried to *make* a heart beat. There was nothing there.

The lioness was *gone*............and I was overcome with the pain of love.

I closed the door to shut out the world. I turned out the light, and for more than an hour I sat sobbing and holding the lioness's limp hand. In that time, and speaking out loud to him, I revealed some regrets. First, he never knew that the mariachis were gone. They never returned after he left home. Second, he never knew he was a lioness. I believe it would have suited him just fine, for he loved the open country. He would have looked very smug.

Tears streamed from my eyes. As sad as it was, nevermore would he roam the Serenghetti, but then again, perhaps he would.

And out of the night, and as plain as day, I could have sworn that I heard the lioness roar.